Effective Health Care Facilities Management

V. James McLarney, General Editor
Linda F. Chaff, Project Editor

for the Division of Health Facilities Management and the American Society for Hospital Engineering of the American Hospital Association

AHA books are published by American Hospital Publishing, Inc., an American Hospital Association company

Library of Congress Cataloging-in-Publication Data

Effective health care facilities management / V. James McLarney,
  general editor ; Linda F. Chaff, project editor ; for the Division
  of Health Facilities Management and the American Society for
  Hospital Engineering of the American Hospital Association.
        p.   cm.
    Includes bibliographical references and index.
    ISBN 1-55648-073-3
      1. Hospitals—Administration—Handbooks, Manuals, etc.
I. McLarney, V. James. II. Chaff, Linda F. III. American Hospital
Association.   Division of Health Facilities Management.
IV. American Society for Hospital Engineering.
  [DNLM: 1. Health Facilities—organization & administration—
handbooks.   WX   39 E27]
RA971.E343   1991
362.1'1'068—dc20
DNLM/DLC
for Library of Congress   91-17196
                                                                              CIP

Catalog no. 055975

Printed in the USA

Text set in Palacio
3M—07/91—0298

Linda Conheady, Marlene Chamberlain, Project Editors
Nancy Charpentier, Editorial Assistant
Marcia Bottoms, Managing Editor
Peggy DuMais, Production Coordinator
Cheryl Kusek, Designer
Brian Schenk, Books Division Director

Contents

List of Figures

List of Tables

Contributors

Nancy Aldrich is vice-president of Computer Task Group's Telecommunications Management Consultants (CTG/TMC), Needham, Massachusetts. Since joining TMC in 1979, Ms. Aldrich has served as a consultant to more than 400 end users including health care institutions, colleges and universities, state and local governments, and private industries and utilities. As a fellow of both the American Society for Hospital Engineering (ASHE) and the Healthcare Information and Management Systems Society (HIMSS), Ms. Aldrich has achieved the highest level of membership awarded for professional and technical competency in the field of health care engineering. She is also a former chairperson of the New England Hospital Telecommunications Association (NEHOSTA). Ms. Aldrich has extensive experience in health care telecommunications and with end users, system manufacturers, and service providers. She has published numerous articles and frequently is a guest speaker at numerous professional organizations.

James Robin Barrick, M.B.A., is president of Smith Seckman Reid, Inc., consulting engineers, in Nashville, where in the past 16 years he has also served as an HVAC design engineer for health care projects, the head of the mechanical department, and a branch office manager. He is currently registered as a professional engineer in 16 states.

Branton B. Blount, P.E., is a facilities engineer at Presbyterian Healthcare Services, Albuquerque, New Mexico. Mr. Blount has had over 30 years' experience in hospital engineering management, including 15 years as director of engineering at Presbyterian Hospital, Dallas, and 12 years with Presbyterian Healthcare Services, Albuquerque, as director of plant services and director of facilities engineering. He is a health care facilities consultant to the state of New Mexico. Mr. Blount has been a member of the American Society for Hospital Engineering for 25 years, serving as president of ASHE in 1985, after having served on the Board of Directors from both Region 7 and Region 8.

Patrick E. Carroll, M.P.H., is vice-president for consulting services with McFaul & Lyons, Inc., a Trenton, New Jersey–based health care consulting firm. He has over 20 years' health care experience and is the immediate past president of the American Society for Hospital Materials Management. He has been involved in a variety of consulting engagements including materials management operations assessments, productivity monitoring, litigation support, strategic planning, revenue enhancement, prospective financial analyses, and general business counseling for all sectors of the health care industry.

Linda F. Chaff is president of Chaff & Co., in Signal Mountain, Tennessee, an organization she founded in 1986 that develops management systems for health care facilities. The company specializes in flexible programs designed to increase company profits and to meet the needs of individual facilities—and individuals. Using a team of people, including technical experts, creative writers, and those with practical experience in the industry, Chaff & Co. develops books, training manuals, and other affordable in-house publications.

For more than 13 years, Ms. Chaff has been actively involved in loss prevention management for the health care industry. She was director of protection services at a 254-bed hospital in West Virginia, where she developed, implemented, and evaluated a comprehensive loss prevention management program.

Her civic involvement includes membership with the American Society for Healthcare Risk Management, the American Society for Training and Development, the National Safety Council's Health Care Section Executive Committee, and the Research and Development Committee for the Safety and Health Hall of Fame. She has also served as a member of the Office of Emergency Services management team in the development of emergency plans and is a certified disaster instructor for the American Red Cross.

Clarence W. Daly, M.H.A., is executive director of the American Society for Healthcare Central Services Personnel, Chicago, a position he has held for over 10 years. Mr. Daly directs and manages the activities of the ASHCSP (a professional organization with over 1,500 members). He develops educational programs and markets the Society and its educational programs, professional activities, and publications. Mr. Daly represents the Society and the American Hospital Association to the Food and Drug Administration and other federal agencies and professional groups that directly affect the area of central service and employee safety. He is an adjunct professor in health care economics at Governors State University.

Douglas S. Erickson is director of design and construction in the Division of Health Facilities Management of the American Hospital Association (AHA), Chicago. In that capacity, he is responsible for health care facilities design, construction, codes and standards, representation and advocacy, educational programming, and technical assistance. Mr. Erickson holds an undergraduate engineering degree and has strong training and experience in the field of facilities management and construction, facilities codes and standards, and the process of planning, designing, and constructing health care facilities. Prior to joining the AHA, Mr. Erickson worked in a number of facilities management positions in large teaching hospitals and was director of engineering for the Joint Commission on Accreditation of Hospitals (now the Joint Commission on Accreditation of Healthcare Organizations). He currently serves on numerous National Fire Protection Association technical committees including NFPA 101, 90A, 70 Panel 17, 110, and is vice-chairman of NFPA 91. Mr. Erickson is also AHA's liaison to other organizations such as the American Institute of Architects's Committee on Architecture for Health, the Joint Commission on Accreditation of Healthcare Organizations, and the model building code organizations.

Jamie C. Kowalski, M.B.A., is president of Kowalski-Dickow Associates, Inc., a Milwaukee-based consulting firm specializing in hospital materials management that has served over 170 hospitals. Mr. Kowalski previously worked in hospital materials management and administration, as well as for a national manufacturer/distributor of hospital products. He has authored dozens of articles, a materials management policy and procedure manual, and has contributed to two other health care management books. He is an editorial board member of *Hospital Materials Management* and a frequent speaker at seminar programs for various health care organizations.

Edward Spivey Lipsey, Jr., P.E., is project manager and mechanical engineer with Smith Seckman Reid, Inc., Nashville. Smith Seckman Reid is a consulting engineering firm specializing in the design of health care facilities.

Carol Hart May, R.D., M.S., D.H.C.F.A., is director of food, nutrition, and environmental services at East Tennessee Baptist Hospital in Knoxville. Her previous experience includes 15 years as director of food and nutrition services at Monongalia General Hospital, Morgantown, West Virginia. She also has been an adjunct professor in the Nutrition and Food Science Department at the University of Tennessee. Ms. May, recognized by the American Society for Hospital Food Service Administrators as a Distinguished Healthcare Food Service Administrator, served on the Board of Directors of ASHFSA for two years.

Sherman G. McGill, Jr., C.P.P., is assistant to the vice-chancellor of facilities and human resources at the University of Tennessee, Memphis. Previously, Mr. McGill served as both director of security/loss prevention and assistant executive director at Eastwood Medical Center, also in Memphis. He has extensive health care security consulting experience and heads Healthtech Security Associates.

V. James McLarney, M.H.A., is director of the Division of Health Facilities Management at the American Hospital Association (AHA) in Chicago. His areas of responsibility include architecture, engineering, safety, security, environmental service, materials management/purchasing, central/sterile supplies, interior design, codes compliance, fire safety, clinical engineering, laundry and linen, and energy management. He manages four AHA personal membership groups—the American Society for Hospital Engineering (ASHE), the American Society for Healthcare Environmental Services (ASHES), the American Society for Hospital Materials Management (ASHMM), and the American Society for Healthcare Central Services Personnel (ASHCSP). Mr. McLarney manages two of the AHA's advocacy program areas, one that deals with environmental issues and another that handles facilities codes and standards. He also manages the AHA's disaster and emergency preparedness efforts as well as health facility compliance services, a consulting service for the AHA. Mr. McLarney serves as contributing editor to *Health Facilities Management* magazine. Mr. McLarney managed clinical laboratories before coming to the AHA.

Hugh O. Nash, Jr., P.E., is senior vice-president of Smith Seckman Reid, Inc., in Nashville, where he is the head of the Healthcare Division. He holds a master's degree in electrical engineering and is licensed to practice electrical engineering in 15 states. He is also a senior member of the Institute of Electrical and Electronics Engineers (IEEE). He is chairman of the IEEE Power Systems Design Subcommittee, chairman of the IEEE White Book Working Group (*Recommended Practice for Electric Systems in Health Care Facilities*), and member of the IEEE Gray Book Working Group (Commercial Buildings). Mr. Nash is also a member of the National Fire Protection Association (NFPA) 70 and NFPA 99 committees and chairman of the NFPA 99 Electrical Systems Subcommittee. He has published 20 technical papers and has received the IEEE Standard Medallion, the IEEE Centennial Medal, and seven IEEE prize paper awards. He has also written and lectured for the American Society for Hospital Engineering.

Sidney Pittman is assistant administrator at West Volusia Memorial Hospital, De Land, Florida. He has been in hospital management since 1965. Mr. Pittman, past president of the American Society for Healthcare Environmental Services, now serves on its board.

Leslie McCall Saunders, A.I.A., is director, medical facilities planning, with Nix, Mann & Associates, an Atlanta architectural firm specializing in hospital planning and design. Mr. Saunders has expertise in medical facilities planning, having planned and designed facilities for over 100 institutions in 16 states and several foreign countries. He is frequently asked to participate on the faculties of regional and national symposia and is a facilitator for institutional retreats.

Aralee Scardina is manager of the Housekeeping Services Department at Saint Luke's Medical Center, in Milwaukee. This 600-bed tertiary care and cardiac center attracts patients, physicians, and students from all over the world. Currently a member of the American Society for Healthcare Environmental Services's Board of Directors, representing Region 5, she has also served as president of the Wisconsin Society for Healthcare Environmental Services. She served on the American Hospital Association's Ad Hoc Committee on Medical Waste and Hazardous Material. She has published articles in environmental services trade journals and written for the Professional Development Series of the American Society for Healthcare Environmental Services. Ms. Scardina has also been a presenter at local and national seminars and workshops.

Gary D. Slack, M.S., is senior consultant for the Management and Compliance Service for the American Hospital Association, Chicago. Mr. Slack has over 14 years' experience in the health care field in the areas of teaching, research, clinical engineering, and management. He is a certified clinical engineer and a registered professional engineer. Mr. Slack has served on various code-making and steering committee panels, written numerous articles related to health facility engineering, and authored two books published by the American Society for Hospital Engineering.

Joseph G. Sprague, A.I.A., is senior vice-president and director of health facilities for HKS Architects, in Dallas. Mr. Sprague has over 20 years' experience in health facilities planning and design. His work has been widely published, and he frequently serves as a consultant, faculty speaker, and lecturer. Prior to joining HKS, he was director of design and construction for the American Hospital Association, where he managed the nationally recognized Health Facility Standards Program and promoted a commonsense approach to facility standards. Mr. Sprague is also past chairman of the Board Health Care Section, National Fire Protection Association, and a member of the Joint Commission on Accreditation of Healthcare Organizations's Committee on Health Care Safety. He also serves on the steering committees of the Planning, Design, and Construction Section of the American Society for Hospital Engineering and the American Institute of Architects's Committee on Architecture for Health.

Preface

The genesis of this book lies in the notion that health facilities management is an area that is taking on renewed importance to health care executives and yet one that receives less than adequate attention in the educational preparation of today's executives. The broad spectrum of health care administration includes such diverse facilities management issues as safety and security, design and construction of new facilities and the renovation of existing structures, central services, environmental services, occupational safety and health, food and nutritional services, energy management, clinical engineering, and the coordination of myriad support services that contribute to a hospital's ability to deliver high-quality patient care. The degree to which health care administrators understand the role of, and effectively manage, their facilities will weigh heavily in their ability to compete and survive in today's health care environment.

Although the value of effective facilities management has not changed in absolute terms, the complexity of the modern health care facility has led to change in the level at which management responsibility is assigned. Over a century ago, top-ranking hospital administrators were referred to as superintendents. These individuals, who may have had greater or lesser roles in planning and managing care, were largely responsible for managing health facilities. The tasks of providing clean linens, potable water, utilities, and materials, as well as the management of housekeeping and maintenance services, grounds keeping, and security, were all under the direction of the hospital superintendent. In addition to certain other important areas, hospital superintendents of that day were responsible for many of the same functions now held by health care facilities managers and/or the heads of the departments described in this book.

As the U.S. health care system continued to evolve, with a host of other issues competing for the attention of the chief executive and with the growth of the *professions* of hospital engineering and other key facility-based managers, health facilities management came less and less to be a part of the management training or the responsibility of health care executives. In the past several decades, however, a variety of forces have led to changes in the health care system, and with those changes have come new demands on those charged with responsibility for facilities management and a renewed importance for understanding and support from top management.

For example, throughout recent history, medical advancements and changes in payment for health care services have led to tremendous growth in the number and nature of outpatient services. As hospitals restructured services vertically and horizontally to respond to changes in technology, demand, and payment, they created a wide variety of new facilities including freestanding outpatient clinics, diagnostic imaging centers, and ambulatory surgicenters, each of which would challenge facilities managers to deal with new building types and new codes and standards. This diversification has also increased the complexity of communication and transportation systems, materials management, security systems, property management, grounds keeping, and all the other facility- and support-related issues.

Other contemporary facilities management issues have their roots in societal change. For example, a growing public awareness and concern for environmental issues have yielded challenges for facilities managers ranging from such relatively simple matters as the choices of cleaning solvents, incineration methods, and disposable products to increasingly more sophisticated institutional programs for occupational health and safety. As a community resource, the health care institution has an obligation to take actions that evidence support for the cause of making a cleaner, safer environment for everyone. As a responsible employer, the health care institution has an obligation to implement and enforce policies regarding global environmental issues.

An issue of immediate concern for hospital administrators is the aging of existing health facilities. Many hospitals have buildings that were constructed decades or many decades ago. Financial and political pressures often deferred attention to needed maintenance and upkeep of buildings and facilities systems. As a result, many hospitals have fallen short of required codes and standards. Although troubled hospitals can often meet pressing operational challenges, Life Safety and other capital-intensive facility codes and standards deficiencies can mark the closing or financial distress for unprepared hospitals. Hospital administrators and boards of directors have an obligation to ensure that the hospital facilities they manage and govern are capable of meeting not only the immediate but also the future needs of their communities.

A shared concern of society and hospitals is the continuous improvement of the quality of health care. Just as clinical staff have a role in identifying actions that will lead to continuous improvements in the quality of patient care, there are facilities management actions that contribute to patient care and the institution's reputation for quality. Patient satisfaction can be enhanced by a well-designed and well-maintained facility, the quality of food service, and the general courteousness and service orientation of all employees.

As the shape of the health care delivery system continues to evolve and consumer-driven issues continue to be a vital and shared concern, administrators can be expected not only to take the ultimate accountability for meeting the needs and challenges of present day-to-day operations but also to plan for the facility's future. For this reason, this book has been designed to aid the health care administrator in understanding the scope of administrative responsibilities of the various departments and functions that come under the umbrella of health facilities management. These responsibilities include:

- The department head's responsibilities
- Staffing within the department
- Specific tasks performed by the department
- Equipment and technology specific to that department
- Specific safety regulations that pertain to the department
- Ways the department evaluates its performance and any product or service it may deliver

Chapters 1 through 4 cover the key departments traditionally defined under the term *facilities management*--engineering and maintenance, clinical engineering, environmental services, and security. Chapters 5 and 6 describe safety and other standards and compliance issues that affect every facility. They also provide information on the governmental agencies and voluntary organizations that affect them. Chapters 7 through 10 describe other departments within a health care facility that may come under the purview of facilities management—telecommunications, materials management, laundry, and food service.

Individuals involved in the construction of new facilities will find helpful information in appendix A, which describes planning considerations and design/construction steps in developing health facility projects. For a perspective on how architecture has influenced health care delivery, appendix B provides background on the architectural history of health care facilities. Appendix C lists organizations that can provide facilities administrators with useful data.

Understanding the scope and concerns of each department within a health care facility, and how each component interrelates to make the facility function as a whole, not only will enable administrators to effectively manage the facility, but also to better compete and survive in today's and tomorrow's health care environment.

V. James McLarney

Acknowledgments

We want to thank the many people who contributed their special talents to this project. Their tireless effort, creativity, and expertise ensured the high quality of this book.

We particularly appreciate the outstanding organizational skills of Marlene Chamberlain, product line manager, American Hospital Publishing, Inc., who set the high standard in the initial phase of the project that the rest of us followed.

We also wish to thank Linda Conheady, assistant managing editor, American Hospital Publishing, Inc., who diligently went through each page with a fine-tooth comb in editing for accuracy and correctness.

The strong foundation of technical content was cemented by the technical expertise of Linda Glasson, Gerald Hengel, John Holcomb, Tony Parente, Gerald Rakes, Dean Samet, Denise Taylor, and Gail Ward through their insightful technical reviews.

Chapter 1

Engineering and Maintenance

Hugh O. Nash, Jr., James Robin Barrick, Edward Spivey Lipsey, Jr., and Branton B. Blount

☐ Overview

The operation and maintenance of the physical plant of a health care facility is the responsibility of the engineering and maintenance department. The physical plant includes the facility's grounds, buildings, mechanical and electrical systems, and equipment. The goal of the engineering and maintenance department is not only to operate the physical plant in an efficient and cost-effective manner, but also to ensure the maximum comfort and safety of the facility's patients, visitors, and staff.

Mechanical systems (including the heating, ventilating, and air-conditioning [HVAC] systems, plumbing, fire protection, and medical gas system) and electrical systems make up about 40 percent of the nonequipment construction cost of a typical new or replacement facility. It is not unusual for these systems to exceed 50 percent of the construction budget for a major hospital remodeling project.

Not only do the mechanical and electrical systems in health care facilities have high initial costs, in terms of energy and maintenance they also have higher operating costs than do such systems in other types of buildings. A typical hospital uses about 275,000 BTUs per square foot per year in energy as compared to a typical office building, which uses about 80,000 BTUs per square foot per year. A typical 300-bed, 400,000-square-foot hospital can have an electric utility bill of over $1 million per year. And HVAC systems have always created more operational and maintenance problems than perhaps any other building system. Additionally, perhaps no other construction type is as closely regulated by federal, state, and local authorities, and no other facility type must comply with as many codes and standards.

It is important for a health care facility to have on staff competent engineering and maintenance personnel who are capable of proficiently operating and maintaining the increasingly complex systems of the modern facility. To understand the importance of the mechanical and electrical systems, one need only consider the systems that support the typical surgical procedure. In addition to controlling the air temperature and humidity of the operating room, HVAC systems provide the proper air circulation and outside air makeup and filtration, and they maintain the pressure relationships required for infection control, all of which are mandated by regulation. Medical gas systems provide oxygen, medical air, and other gases for life support and anesthesia, and vacuum systems provide critical support functions. Other mechanical systems safely remove exhausted anesthesia gases and contaminated air. Electrical systems provide safe electric power, including proper grounding and special systems for protecting patients and staff from electric shock. Emergency power systems stand ready to provide power in the event of a utility outage or an internal hospital power failure. Certainly, it is no wonder that modern hospitals require well-designed, properly installed, proficiently operated, and well-maintained mechanical and electrical systems in order for the medical staff to properly treat patients.

The general maintenance of equipment, buildings, and grounds is also very important to patients, visitors, and staff, especially in terms of the facility's appearance. This chapter discusses the responsibilities, problems, and issues of the department's operation in general and focuses on those of the department head and supervisory staff in particular.

☐ Department Head Responsibilities

The head of the engineering and maintenance department may be known as Director of Plant Services, Director of Engineering (or of Engineering and Maintenance), Plant Engineer, Facilities Engineer, Physical Plant Manager, Manager of Engineering Services, or other similar titles that denote the technical responsibilities of this position. The engineer who is the department head (hereafter called the director) has the overall responsibility for the proper operation and maintenance of the facility's physical plant. The director is also responsible for setting the goals and standards of the department, as well as preparing the budget for the physical plant's operation and maintenance.

Depending on the size of the facility and the size of the engineering and maintenance staff, the director may supply all or most of the engineering and technical support for the department and for the facility as a whole. If there are assistant department heads or division directors, the director may delegate the daily responsibilities for the operation of the physical plant.

Health care facilities utilize some of the more complex and technical mechanical and electrical systems found in modern buildings and contain numerous pieces of highly technical and sensitive diagnostic and treatment equipment. Because of this, facilities of about 100 beds or more usually require that the director of the engineering and maintenance department have five or more years' supervisory experience in such a department, together with an engineering degree, usually either mechanical or electrical.

☐ Staffing

As with the staffing in most health care facility departments, the staffing of the engineering and maintenance department is directly related to the size of the facility. The number of operating and maintenance staff members in the department depends on a number of factors, including the licensing requirements of the city, county, or state in which the facility is located, as well as the facility's size and complexity.

In smaller facilities of 50 beds or fewer, usually two or three general maintenance people report directly to the director. In larger facilities, an assistant department head and two or more supervisors can divide the responsibilities for plant operation and maintenance.

In still larger facilities, having several hundred beds or more, the management team of the department might consist of the director, an associate department head, and assistant department heads for plant operations and maintenance, with one or more supervisors reporting to each assistant. As the size of the facility increases, so do the sophistication and complexity of its mechanical and electrical systems. As a result, these systems require managers and operating and maintenance personnel who are more technically qualified.

Contract Services

Some health care facilities contract out either all or part of their engineering and maintenance functions. Contract services may be obtained from either locally owned and operated firms or nationally known ones.

As with most contracted work, there are advantages and disadvantages. Although most contract firms operate similarly to in-house departments, they may have access to additional management tools or special computer programs. Although contract services may offer certain cost advantages, there may be trade-offs in quality and commitment for the long-term well-being of the facility. Other considerations include control of both personnel and management prerogatives. Many facilities have found an effective balance by having general in-house services and using contract services for highly sophisticated technologies and equipment.

For grounds maintenance, for example, some facilities find it more cost-effective to have an experienced grounds maintenance supervisor with a small crew, supplemented by temporary "summer hires" during the peak growing season. Because of the relatively seasonal nature of this work (and the visibility of the results), as well as the competitiveness of the contractors, grounds maintenance is contracted out more often than other tasks performed by the department.

If maintenance personnel are not technically qualified to work on a certain piece of equipment, this work would be contracted to an outside service firm. Employees should be trained to know which equipment is serviced in-house and which is contracted out.

☐ Specific Tasks Done within the Department

The primary objective of the department is to operate the mechanical and electrical systems of the physical plant so that patients, visitors, and staff have a safe and comfortable environment. To accomplish this, there are several tasks that enable the department to run in the most efficient and cost-effective manner possible:

- *Preventive maintenance programs:* These include monitoring equipment to ensure proper performance, reviewing equipment incident history, and documenting scheduled service and repairs.
- *Building maintenance:* This includes repairing or adjusting door latches and closures, painting and repairing walls, changing light bulbs, and repairing equipment.
- *Grounds maintenance:* This includes providing attractive, well-maintained lawns, trees, and plantings; providing a snow removal service; performing indoor tasks during inclement weather (for example, cleaning mechanical rooms or remodeling areas); and assisting the preventive maintenance crew.

The engineering function also includes providing in-house engineering support and consultation to administration and other departments. Additionally, during the design stage of additions or new facilities the department works closely with the operating and design engineers regarding the design of new systems. It is important to combine the expertise of both the facility engineer and the design engineer.

☐ Equipment and Technology

Over the past several decades, a number of tremendous technological developments have had considerable impact on the mechanical and electrical systems of health care facilities.

To understand some of the issues and complexities faced in satisfying the design requirements for mechanical and electrical systems, a description of the various types of systems used in health care facilities follows.

Mechanical Systems

The mechanical systems of a health care facility include the heating, ventilating, and air-conditioning (HVAC) systems; domestic cold and hot water; steam for sterilization, cooking, heating, and humidification; heating hot water; sanitary and storm sewers; medical gas systems; transport systems such as pneumatic tube and conveyor systems; fire pump and sprinkler systems; and vacuum systems. The proper design, installation, operation, and maintenance of these systems are critical because they all contribute to patient care, comfort, and safety.

There is no one best system or combination of systems available to meet the needs of every facility. Before the selection is finalized, a number of factors should be considered. These include code and environmental requirements, operation and maintenance characteristics, budget constraints, and personal preference.

The following sections describe some of the mechanical systems commonly used in health care facilities. The functions, advantages, and disadvantages of each system are also discussed.

Hospital Air-Handling Systems

The heating, ventilating, and air-conditioning (HVAC) systems in a health care facility provide the interior environment required for safety, comfort, and patient care by maintaining filtration, pressurization, and comfortable temperatures and relative humidity (figure 1-1).

Health care facilities differ from most other types of facilities in that their requirements for filtration, temperature, and humidity control are far more critical because their occupants are sick and immobile. Health care codes and standards recognize the critical nature of the environment within health care facilities and provide specific requirements for temperature, humidity, filtration, pressure relationships, and outside air ventilation for the various patient care areas. Typical requirements for these various criteria are shown in table 1-1.

Figure 1-1. Functions of the HVAC System

1. Heating and cooling to maintain the temperature in individual areas at a comfortable level, usually between 72° F and 76° F, depending on the function of the area served and applicable codes and standards.
2. Dehumidification or humidification to maintain the relative humidity at a comfortable level, normally between 40 percent and 60 percent, again depending on the function of the area and applicable codes and standards.
3. Introduction of outside air to remove carbon dioxide and chemicals from building components, and to dilute odors.
4. Filtration of both outside air and air recirculated within the building to provide a clean environment.
5. Provision of air motion within the rooms, which enhances the evaporation of perspiration and a feeling of comfort.
6. Maintenance of air pressure relationships between adjacent areas to prevent contamination of clean areas. In the case of isolation rooms (and depending on the type of isolation required), provision of either positive or negative pressure relative to adjacent areas.
7. Pressurization of the building to minimize undesirable infiltration of outside air at doors and windows, which can create hot or cold drafts.
8. Pressurization of certain areas of the building in the event of fire or smoke to prevent smoke from moving from one smoke compartment to another. Some systems also provide a smoke purge system, in which the air-handling systems serving an affected area provide full outside air and full exhaust to prevent the recirculation of smoke and to purge the smoke from the building.

Table 1-1. Filter Efficiencies for Central Ventilation and Air-Conditioning Systems in General Hospitals

Area Designation	Number of Filter Beds	Filter Efficiencies (percent)	
		Filter Bed No. 1	Filter Bed No. 2
All areas for inpatient care, treatment, and/or diagnosis and those areas providing direct service or clean supplies, such as laboratories, sterile and clean processing, and so on	2	25	90
Food preparation areas and laundries	1	80	—
Administrative, bulk storage, and soiled holding areas	1	25	—

Source: U.S. Department of Health and Human Services Publication No. (HRS-M-HF) 84-1, *Guidelines for Construction and Equipment of Hospital and Medical Facilities*, copyright 1987 The American Institute of Architects. Reprinted with permission under license number 91052.

Note: Ratings shall be based on American Society of Heating, Refrigerating, and Air-Conditioning Engineers Standard 52-76.

HVAC System Types

The American Society of Heating, Refrigerating, and Air-Conditioning Engineers (ASHRAE) divides the various HVAC systems into four general classifications: all-air systems, air-and-water systems, all-water systems, and packaged-unitary systems. The classifications are based on how the cooling capacity is delivered and controlled.

1. *All-air systems* deliver all their cooling capacity in the cold air supplied by the system, with heating accomplished in the same manner. Control of the temperature in particular spaces is by either varying the volume of the cold and/or warm air discharged into the space or controlling the flow of warm water in the reheat coil (see figure 1-2).

   The principal advantages of all-air systems are that the centralized location of the air-handling unit permits ease of maintenance of the equipment; no condensate drain lines, electrical power, or filters are required in the air-conditioned space; and there is the greatest potential for use of outdoor air for cooling instead of mechanical refrigeration. Among the disadvantages are the additional space requirements for the larger air duct, the difficulty in balancing the air in certain systems, and the fact that all-air reheat systems are very energy inefficient.

2. *Air-and-water systems* deliver cooling capacity using air-and-water sources supplied from a central location and distributed to terminal units located in the air-conditioned space. The terminals generally used in this type of system are induction units and fan-coil units. With induction units, the air supplied to the unit from the central air-handling unit induces additional air from the space to flow through the water coil, which adds the additional cooling or heating capacity to satisfy the thermostat setting (see figure 1-3). The same quantity of air supplied by the central unit is then exhausted from the space to provide the required ventilation. With fan-coil units, the conditioned air from the central unit is either ducted directly to the return air of the fan-coil unit or discharged directly into the air-conditioned space, with an equal quantity being exhausted to balance the system.

   Some of the advantages of air-and-water systems are that individual room temperature can be easily controlled (for example, when the weather is mild, the occupant can select either heating or cooling); less duct space is required; and the size of the central unit is smaller. The disadvantages are that the design is more critical due to the smaller quantity of air, especially in fall and winter; the

Figure 1-2. **Example of an All-Air System**

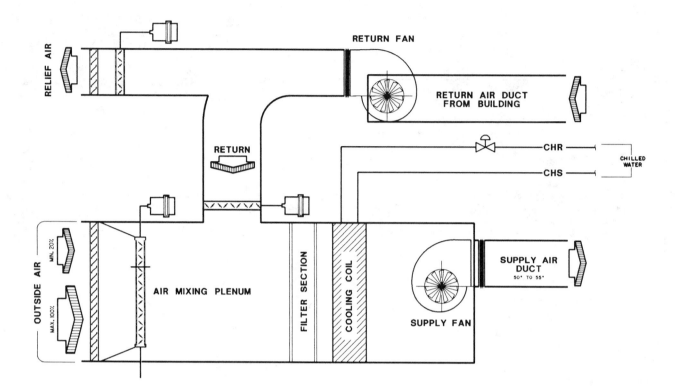

Figure 1-3. **Example of an Air-and-Water System**

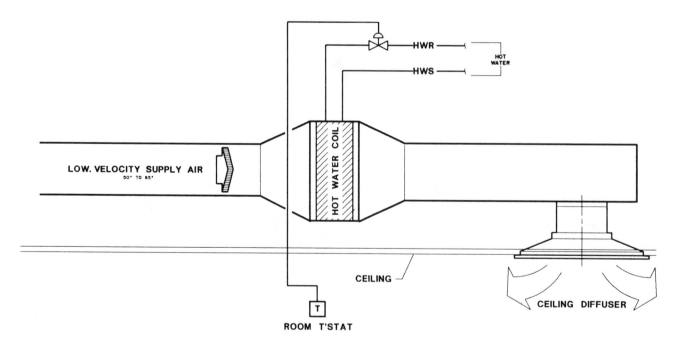

induction system has operating complexities not common to other systems; the primary air supply is constant, with no provision for shutoff of individual units; and application is limited to the perimeter space of the building.

3. *All-water systems* provide space cooling by circulating chilled water from the central refrigeration system through the cooling coils in the terminal units located in the conditioned space. The terminal units are usually fan-coil units or unit ventilators, located above the ceiling or on the outside walls under windows. Heating is accomplished by circulating hot water in the same or parallel coil in the terminal unit. Ventilation is supplied through either a ducted system or vents in the wall to the outside.

The advantages of the system are that the building space is reduced because of reduced central fan room space and duct space requirements; the units allow for individual room control and shutoff; and there is no recirculated air between spaces, with no cross-contamination.

The disadvantages are that all-water systems require more maintenance than all-air systems; maintenance must be done in the occupied space; and each unit requires a condensate drain.

4. *Packaged-unitary systems* are basically individual air-conditioning units manufactured in various configurations such as window units, through-the-wall units, rooftop units, and heat pumps. Although these units are applied in all types of buildings, they are especially applicable where performance is less demanding, initial cost is important, and installation is simple.

The advantages are that individual room control is inexpensive; heating and cooling can be provided at all times independent of other rooms; and the failure of one unit affects only that unit. The disadvantages are that the available options are limited as to size and capacity; units are not suited for close humidity control; thermostat action is usually on/off, causing temperature swings; and energy and maintenance costs are usually higher.

Central Plant Equipment

In most facilities, a strong case can be made for locating all the major mechanical and electrical equipment in a central energy center. This equipment includes boilers, chillers, water softeners, domestic hot-water heaters, fire pumps, emergency generators, electrical service entrance, transformers, and switchboards, as well as gas and water services. Ideally, the facility's clinical air compressor and vacuum pumps would also be located in the central energy center. There are several advantages to having a centrally located energy center containing the aforementioned equipment, which include:

- Lower initial costs, because the incremental costs per unit of capacity decrease as the equipment size increases
- Lower operating costs, because larger equipment generally has a higher operating efficiency than smaller equipment
- Increase in patient safety, because fuel-burning equipment is located away from patient care areas
- Reduction in operating and maintenance costs
- Longer service life and therefore a lower life cycle cost
- Reduction in the capital cost of implementing future energy-saving measures, such as cogeneration and heat recovery
- Reduction in the noise level throughout the facility

Boilers
Boilers usually burn either natural gas or fuel oil to produce steam at pressures between 65 and 125 pounds per square inch. Normally, if the boilers burn natural gas, they are

also equipped to burn fuel oil as a backup in the event that gas service is curtailed for some reason.

Health care facility standards require that at least two boilers be maintained in the event that one malfunctions. Requirements also specify that the boiler plant be capable of providing steam for heating, sterilization, and cooking. Many plants will have three boilers, with the smallest one used in warm weather to save energy and increase operating efficiency.

The steam produced by the boilers is used to provide the following services:

- Space heating within the facility
- Domestic hot-water heating
- Humidification
- Sterilization
- Booster heaters for kitchen dishwashers
- Steam supply to dietary equipment, such as steam kettles and pressure cookers
- Steam supply to flatwork ironers, washers, and dryers in facilities with an in-house laundry

Chillers

In health care facilities with a central chilled-water plant that supplies chilled water to central station air-handling units or fan-coil units, the chillers are usually located in the central energy plant and the water is pumped through a system of pipes to and from these units. The chillers are usually one of the following types: electric drive centrifugal, reciprocating, steam or direct-gas-fired absorption, or screw drive.

The electric drive centrifugal water chiller is usually the most efficient and reliable choice for a central chilled-water plant. Reciprocating chillers, which compress the refrigerant using a reciprocating piston, have more moving parts and are less reliable. However, they may be used for very small loads because they can be purchased with a much smaller capacity than centrifugal machines.

The absorption machine uses steam, high-temperature hot water, or direct-gas firing to produce chilled water for the facility. In this system, a lithium bromide brine is evaporated and reconcentrated in the absorption cycle to produce chilled water. It is not a very energy-efficient system when compared to the electric-drive machines. However, to the extent absorption chillers can be driven by excess or waste heat from either cogeneration or discharge from a steam-driven turbine, savings can be realized and the system considered a viable alternative.

The screw-drive machine operates much like the centrifugal machine, except that the refrigerant is compressed by means of a screw rotating in a cylinder rather than by a large centrifugal impellor. The screw machine is comparable in cost and operating characteristics to a centrifugal machine, and it offers another possible advantage: It has the ability to produce colder water or a colder brine solution, which would allow a thermal ice storage type of system to be used in the facility. Thus cooling capacity could be generated and stored during off-peak hours (usually at night) at a lower electrical rate and utilized during the peak air-conditioning load period, reducing the operating cost.

There has been much discussion recently about types of refrigerants and the greenhouse warming effect, and ozone layer damage caused by the venting of these refrigerants, typically chlorofluorocarbons, into the atmosphere. Because of these issues, manufacturers are beginning to seek alternative refrigerant types and change their equipment to allow less harmful refrigerants to be used.

Energy Conservation Methods

Energy conservation was a hot topic in the late 1970s and early 1980s. Owners of buildings of every type implemented many energy-saving measures, regardless of cost, for fear of exorbitant prices and curtailed availability of fuel.

As budgets tighten and saving every energy dollar becomes more important, health care facilities are once again looking for ways to save energy. Today, however, energy-saving methods must be evaluated on the initial cost as well as the annual savings potential to determine the most effective measures from a cost–payback standpoint. The greatest savings from energy conservation efforts (up to 20 percent) often come from low-cost operating and maintenance improvements.

These low-cost measures include such strategies as high-efficiency lighting, strict maintenance of steam traps and other components of high-energy-using systems, appropriate sizing of motors and pumps, attention to the temperature settings of hot water and heating/cooling systems, and so forth.

Any energy management program should begin with an "audit" of how and where savings might be realized. A walk-through evaluation of the facility by technically prepared staff can reveal valuable opportunities that can produce immediate savings.

When all low-cost opportunities have been exhausted, an evaluation of capital opportunities should be conducted. This evaluation is often conducted by an external engineering firm specializing in energy management. The prioritized recommendations of this effort should be incorporated into the hospital's capital acquisition process and implemented according to their ability to contribute to the financial well-being of the facility.

The most common energy conservation methods in health care facilities rest in modifications to the HVAC system. Examples are air-side economizers, water-side economizers, and heat recovery from either heat sources such as incinerators or exhausted air. Air-side economizers involve utilizing outside air for cooling when the ambient temperature is low enough.

Because nearly all health care facilities have areas that require year-round cooling, a water-side economizer can effectively cool without using mechanical refrigeration during certain times of the year and under certain ambient conditions. When a building or portions of a building require a chilled-water supply during periods of the year when the outdoor wet bulb temperature (relative humidity) is low, chilled water can be produced by using a cooling tower in lieu of mechanical refrigeration. The savings come from eliminating the compressor motor from the cooling process. A water-side economizer uses the condenser water from the cooling tower and passes it through a heat exchanger where it cools down or chills water for the building's air-conditioning. When conditions are too hot outside for a water-side economizer to work effectively, the chilled water simply bypasses the heat exchanger and flows through a mechanical refrigeration machine or *chiller*, where it is cooled.

Heat recovery (for example, heat exchange) has been utilized as an energy conservation method for a number of years. This method simply exchanges heat between the air exhausts of the facility and the air intakes by run-around coils, heat wheels, or refrigerant pipes. The concept is to preheat fresh-air intake in the winter by transferring otherwise wasted heat from the exhaust air to it. Similarly, the fresh-air intake in the summer months is precooled by extracting heat from that air and discharging it into the exhaust air. The net effect is to reduce the heating and cooling loads because of ventilation.

Other heat recovery methods include the recovery of heat from the incineration of solid waste generated by the facility. Although this is a viable method of energy conservation, the wide variance in state and local laws controlling the use of incinerators and emissions from them has squelched enthusiasm for committing funds for new incinerator facilities. Justification for incineration and associated heat recovery methods must be investigated individually and to a great extent depends on local regulations.

Electrical Systems

Over the past several decades, the electrical loads of lighting and equipment systems in health care facilities have increased dramatically. Along with the overall increase, the loads on the essential electrical system, serving the critical life safety systems and lighting and equipment essential to maintaining patient care during emergency conditions, also increased.

The principal requirements of the electrical system in a health care facility are reliability, quality, and safety. These factors are all important whether in the design, installation, or operation of the facility's electrical systems. However, they are especially important at the design stage.

The particular requirements for the electrical power systems, as opposed to the alarm, control, and communication systems, are spelled out in chapter 3, Electrical Systems, of the National Fire Protection Association (NFPA) 99 Healthcare Facilities Standards. Usually, the facility receives its normal power service from an electrical utility. In the event of an electric utility service interruption, the facility provides on-site emergency generators to maintain electrical power to the essential electrical system.

To deliver reliable electric power to the end-use load, no matter how remotely located in the facility, four things are required:

1. A reliable primary, or normal, source of power, usually an electric utility
2. A reliable standby generator and essential electrical system
3. A well-designed distribution system with adequate and coordinated protective devices
4. An adequate number of receptacles in the patient care areas, conveniently placed, properly grounded, and connected to the facility's normal or essential electrical systems

Normal Power

The normal power for a health care facility is usually supplied by the electric utility serving the area. Whenever possible, the facility should be served by a dual electrical service. This service can be accomplished in several ways depending, to a large extent, on the rules or policies of the utility. Some utilities furnish the additional service, with the health care facility furnishing a manual or automatic transfer device. Still others furnish the entire dual service at no additional charge as a community service, although this is not the usual case.

To be effective, a dual service should be fed from different branches of the utility's distribution system, preferably from two separate substations. The facility should evaluate whether the offered secondary service is truly separate and independent from the primary service. The reliability of the utility's system should also be evaluated.

Standby Power and Essential Electrical Systems

Although overall electrical system reliability is important, it is the essential electrical system that ensures the reliability of the surgeon's operating light, the anesthesiologist's patient monitoring equipment, and the patient's ventilator in ICU, as well as the operation of all vital electrical equipment, lighting, and systems.

NFPA 99, paragraph 3-3, outlines specific requirements for both normal and alternate sources of power. The standard subdivides the essential electrical system into two separate systems: equipment system and emergency system. The equipment system supplies mechanical equipment used to support patient care. The standard is quite specific about which pieces of mechanical equipment are to be served by the equipment system. Items include heating for critical areas and patient rooms; clinical air compressors and vacuum pumps; air systems with special air change, filtration, or pressurization requirements; and other equipment such as sterilizers, elevators, and sump pumps.

The emergency system includes the critical and life safety branches. The critical branch generally serves patient care areas, life support systems, anesthetizing areas, and other electrical loads essential for patient care and medical staff support. The life safety branch serves egress and exit lighting, fire alarm systems, and other systems required for the life safety of the patient, staff, and public.

Life Safety

Health care facilities deal with fires and other life-threatening emergencies differently from other building types (such as offices, schools, or factories). In most building types, the objective is to evacuate the occupants as rapidly as possible. In hospitals, the objective is to "protect in place." The strategy is to notify the fire department (usually by automatic means) and the staff of the emergency, relocate any patient endangered by the fire to a safe area on the same floor, and then contain and suppress the fire. Total evacuation or discontinuing certain medical procedures, such as surgery, is usually out of the question.

Patient Electrical Safety

The design of electrical systems for buildings includes certain features for the protection of occupants, the public, and maintenance personnel. In general, the strategy includes protecting people from energized or live parts and grounding metallic surfaces likely to become energized. Grounding is achieved by means of metallic conduit and raceway systems as well as by grounding conductors installed in conduits with the supply conductors.

Grounding accomplishes two things. First, it provides a low-resistance or low-impedance return path for fault or short circuit currents, and thus ensures that fault currents are of sufficient magnitude to cause circuit breakers to trip and fuses to blow, de-energizing the grounded object. Second, grounding ensures that metallic surfaces likely to become energized and come in contact with a person, such as in the case of portable electrical equipment, remain at ground potential or at the same voltage as the earth or floor on which the person is standing.

In addition to the usual concern for staff, the public, and maintenance personnel, hospitals must be even more concerned with the electrical safety of patients. Hospital patients are at times particularly vulnerable to electric shock because:

- Patients are exposed to, and even connected to, a variety of electrical equipment.
- Patients are often catheterized with conductive electrical and nonelectrical catheters that penetrate the skin, which is the body's natural high-resistance barrier to electric shock.
- Patients are often anesthetized or sedated and thus rendered less alert to their surroundings.

The protective systems and equipment designed to protect patients, staff, and maintenance personnel are spelled out by the various regulatory agencies and include grounding requirements for equipment, special grounding conductors, ground fault circuit interrupting receptacles in wet locations, isolated power systems in "wet" anesthetizing locations, and regular testing of these systems as well as leakage testing of patient care equipment. All these requirements were designed to eliminate or at least minimize the possibility of electric shock.

☐ Safety and Compliance

Virtually all the various tasks performed by the engineering and maintenance department involve safety, either directly or indirectly. The department is responsible for its own departmental safety program, including training and monitoring the work practices of departmental personnel, correcting unsafe conditions throughout the facility and grounds, and maintaining and testing fire safety systems.

To better coordinate the correction and evaluation of reported unsafe conditions, the departmental director should represent the department on the facility safety committee. The safety of patients, visitors, and staff should be of prime importance to the engineering and maintenance department. Additionally, this issue is stressed as an important aspect of operations in the Joint Commission on Accreditation of Healthcare Organizations's (Joint Commission's) Plant Technology and Safety Management Standards, as well as in the licensing regulations of many states.

The engineering and maintenance department is directly responsible for compliance with the applicable fire safety regulations. The department's management team must keep abreast of the latest changes in or additions to those codes and regulations that are enforced by the various regulatory agencies. For example, all health care facilities are required to comply with specific health care facilities standards of the National Fire Protection Association (NFPA). These codes are enforced by several agencies, including state licensing agencies, the Health Care Financing Administration (HCFA), and state and local fire marshals. Associations such as the Joint Commission also advocate standards. Compliance with a particular edition may vary from state to state, depending on the latest edition that has been adopted by the particular agency.

In addition, certain states and cities have adopted either their own fire code or one of the three Model Building Codes. Many times, there are conflicting requirements in the various codes used to inspect the same facility.

Another nationwide code that must be complied with is NFPA 70, the National Electrical Code. Although it primarily applies to new construction, specific sections do apply to remodeling. In the case of NFPA 101, the Life Safety Code, chapters adopted in the sections on existing facilities are retroactively enforceable when the edition is adopted.

Still another nationwide standard is NFPA 99, the Health Care Facilities Standard, whose format is patterned after that of the Life Safety Code. The requirements are spelled out in the "occupancy" chapters and the "how to comply" sections in the early chapters. Whereas NFPA 101 covers the fire safety construction requirements for the facility, NFPA 99 addresses the systems requirements for particular areas in the facility.

Perhaps the most important compliance survey or inspection of a health care facility is the accreditation survey for eligibility to receive Medicare and Medicaid funds. A survey performed by either the Joint Commission or one of the various state licensing agencies may form the basis for Medicare and Medicaid eligibility. Occasionally a follow-up survey by HCFA is required. Although the Joint Commission and these agencies do develop particular standards on their own, the majority of their standards are based on (or include by direct reference) the standards of the NFPA. In addition to NFPA 101, NFPA 70, and NFPA 99, as discussed above, the standards include a number of other NFPA standards such as the NFPA 72 (series) on fire alarms, detectors, and signaling systems; NFPA 80, Fire Doors and Windows; NFPA 90A, Air Conditioning and Ventilating Systems; NFPA 110, Emergency and Standby Power Systems; and NFPA 13, Sprinkler Systems.

The department must also comply with various Occupational Safety and Health Administration regulations, including an ongoing right-to-know program regarding precautions to be taken by departmental personnel when using certain hazardous chemicals.

If the department operates an incinerator, it must operate, maintain, and monitor the incinerator in accordance with state and local regulations regarding emissions. In older facilities, the department is responsible for any asbestos abatement programs that may become necessary.

Furthermore, facilities must manage any buried fuel oil tanks not only supplying their emergency generators but being used as back-up fuel for natural gas–fired boilers as well.

In addition to all the codes and regulations just discussed, the department is responsible for compliance with state and local building, plumbing, and mechanical codes.

However, its involvement with these codes is generally limited to the renovation and remodeling of the facility.

☐ Program Evaluation

The ultimate beneficiary of the proficient operation of the department is the patient. In a very real sense, the department provides the physical environment necessary for the facility's medical, nursing, treatment, diagnostic, and support staff to perform their best work on the patient's behalf.

There are many ways that excellent performance by the engineering and maintenance department supports and even enhances patient care. Examples of this could include the repeatedly reliable operation of patient care equipment, reliable emergency back-up power, the provision of stable and comfortable environmental conditions for the operating room, and the assurance of the administration that the physical plant and systems are performing as they should and at peak cost-effectiveness.

Insofar as patient care is concerned, quality assurance (QA) has been a primary focus of health care facilities for the past decade or more, given impetus by the emphasis placed on it by the Joint Commission. Although the Joint Commission has essentially limited its emphasis to departments providing direct patient care, the inclusion of all the facility's departments under an overall QA program is already a reality in some facilities. Because the engineering and maintenance department's performance has such a profound effect on the environment of the health care facility, it is very important that the department design an operational program for systematically evaluating the department's objectives and goals.

In the American Society for Hospital Engineering Technical Document Series article titled "Quality Assurance for the Hospital Engineering/Maintenance Department" (1989), David Sheets defines *quality assurance* for the department as follows: "In short, quality assurance is more than simply retrospectively evaluating data and making reports; it is a concentrated effort of evaluation that should be aimed at improving (or proving) quality of service." He states that the same degree of excellence expected of clinicians when providing patient care should be part of the engineering/maintenance function. In placing their lives and comfort in the hands of the health care facility, patients expect nothing less than excellence of care and trust that they will receive it.

An effective departmental QA program provides management with the tool that it needs to evaluate the quality and effectiveness of its operations. This process should be accomplished through the active involvement of the management team, along with the encouraged participation of departmental personnel. The department's QA program should be coordinated with the facilitywide program which, as Sheets so aptly concludes, "demonstrates the relationship of the department to patient care, and emphasizes the important treatment tools health professionals have . . . the physical plant and equipment."

☐ Summary

The engineering and maintenance department is responsible for providing and maintaining the physical environment required for excellence in patient care. For the department to fulfill its responsibility to the facility, and ultimately to the patient, it must have experienced, competent engineering employees. These individuals should not only understand system technologies and how to operate them efficiently, but also understand the operations of each department within the facility. With competent management and well-trained operation and maintenance personnel, the department should be capable of addressing the many operational and maintenance problems that continually occur, as well as achieve the optimization desired.

Although the engineering and maintenance department does not deal directly with patient care in the facility, virtually every aspect of the department's operation has some indirect effect on the care of the facility's patients, visitors, and staff. In effect, it provides the physical environment that supports the efforts of the health care professionals to provide excellent care to the patients.

☐ References and Bibliography

American Society of Heating, Refrigerating, and Air-Conditioning Engineers, Inc. *American Society of Heating, Refrigerating, and Air-Conditioning Engineers Handbook, 1984 Systems Volume.* Atlanta: ASHRAE, 1984.

National Fire Protection Association. *NFPA 99: Health Care Facilities Standard, 1987 edition.* Quincy, MA: NFPA, 1987.

National Fire Protection Association. *NFPA 101 Life Safety Code.* 1985 ed. Quincy, MA: NFPA, 1985.

Sheets, D. *Quality Assurance for the Hospital Engineering/Maintenance Department.* Technical Document Series No. 055925. Chicago: American Society for Hospital Engineering, Nov. 1989.

Chapter 2
Clinical Engineering

Gary D. Slack

☐ Overview

As a department within the health care facility, clinical engineering is relatively new. Prior to World War II, technology in even the most advanced health care facility was limited to single-tube X-ray units, spark-gap cautery devices, fragile electrocardiograph machines, and an assortment of vacuum and compressor-driven suction pumps. Repair of these devices was usually performed as needed by the mechanic or electrician within the facility's maintenance department. Often, little attention was given to performance or potential patient liability. Usually, the physicians or nursing staff determined whether a piece of equipment was safe or unsafe for patient treatment.

Beginning in the late 1950s, and continuing throughout the 1960s, several significant trends began to develop. Technological devices and equipment that were being developed for use in the space program began to find applications in the health care field. The concept of electrically monitoring the vital signs of patients gained acceptance. With the refinement of solid-state electronics, health care diagnostic and treatment equipment became smaller, lighter, and more reliable, although maintenance and repair of the equipment was still necessary.

A major event occurred in 1969 that had a tremendous impact on the growth and development of the clinical engineering field. At a meeting of surgeons, Dr. Carl Walter concluded that thousands of patients annually were being accidentally electrocuted in hospitals (Walter, 1970). Although conclusive evidence had not yet been obtained, Ralph Nader, who was an active consumer advocate at the time, brought public attention to this issue by claiming that at least 1,200 patients were being electrocuted in hospitals each year (Nader, 1971). Suddenly, the race was on to create a safe electrical environment within hospitals.

Figure 2-1 provides a time-line summary of the historical development of clinical technology that has in turn had an impact on the development of clinical engineering. Throughout the past two decades, clinical engineering departments have gained acceptance not only as a necessary support service within the health care facility, but also as a department that influences risk management, purchasing, and patient treatment effectiveness.

Figure 2-1. Historical Development of Clinical Technology

Decade	Development
1920s	Electrocardiograph machines used to record patient heart signals Use of X-rays for patient radiographs Invention of spark-gap generator for use in electrosurgery
1940s	Widespread use of anesthesia machines and compression pumps during surgery
1960s	Patient monitoring during surgery and for critically ill patients Proliferation of electromedical devices in the hospital
1970s	Electrical safety "scare" and widespread adoption of electrical safety standards by Joint Commission, NFPA, AAMI Expansion of clinical engineering programs to meet increasing demands of equipment testing, repair, and application
1980s	Continued growth of diagnostic and treatment devices including lasers, lithotripsy, magnetic resonance imagers, and sophisticated patient monitoring systems
1990s	Transition of clinical engineering department into technology management service

The following data will help illustrate the necessity of having clinical engineering expertise available to the modern health care facility: In 1980, an average acute care community health care facility could expect to have equipment inventories of approximately 1.5 patient diagnostic or treatment devices per occupied bed. In just 10 years, that ratio increased to nearly seven devices per occupied bed (Slack, 1991). It is estimated that the presence of patient-related equipment will continue to grow in the future.

Although facility administrators often assume that the primary function of the clinical engineering department is to test and repair patient equipment, the department plays other roles as well. Important responsibilities of the department include in-service training, consultation with clinical and ancillary staff, environmental testing, and incident or product recall investigations that involve patient diagnostic or treatment equipment. These specific responsibilities will be described later in this chapter.

☐ Clinical Engineering Terms

Because the term *clinical engineering* is used to describe many different functions, it is necessary to define several common terms to fully comprehend the scope of the department. Clinical engineering is sometimes called biomedical engineering.

The term *clinical engineering* describes the activity that applies engineering technology within a clinical patient care setting such as a health care facility. A *clinical engineer* is someone who, through sufficient training and experience, is able to provide information to the clinical staff concerning the diagnostic and treatment devices and equipment within the facility. In major health care facilities, university medical centers, and specialized acute care clinics, one or more full-time clinical engineers are typically hired to provide technical management and departmental leadership.

Engineers who possess similar training, but apply their knowledge to research endeavors, are called *biomedical engineers* and are typically employed by research laboratories or academic institutions.

A third group, called *medical engineers,* use their training and experience to design equipment that is intended to be used for patient diagnosis and treatment. Usually, these professionals are employed by large medical equipment manufacturers. Electrocardiograph (ECG) monitors, magnetic resonance imagers (MRIs), and computerized axial tomography (CAT) scanners are several examples of the technology and equipment that medical engineers have developed.

Within clinical engineering departments there are usually one or more *biomedical equipment technicians* (BMETs) whose primary function is to test, calibrate, maintain, and repair the clinical equipment. Entry-level positions within a facility usually require at least a two-year degree in biomedical equipment technology. Often, internship programs are provided to these technicians prior to graduation.

In hospitals with fewer than 300 beds, the clinical engineering department frequently consists of technicians only. Engineering expertise is usually obtained as needed from outside consulting services. Figure 2-2 describes the terms used, areas of employment, and functions for the engineers and technicians employed in these four areas of biomedical technology.

☐ Department Head Responsibilities

In addition to providing leadership within the department, clinical engineering directors have other responsibilities that enhance the department's overall operation:

- *Preparing periodic management reports:* The clinical engineering supervisor or department manager is accountable for reporting staff productivity (at least an activity analysis), changes in equipment inventory, and effectiveness in performing job responsibilities. The report should be integrated with the facilitywide quality assurance program so that meaningful monitoring indicators are used.
- *Establishing a separate cost center for clinical engineering:* Even if the clinical engineering function is assigned within the maintenance department, the facility should consider establishing separate budgets. When attempting to compare costs for outside versus in-house services, it is essential that accurate financial data be available to determine the preventive maintenance and repair cost for specific devices.

Figure 2-2. Areas of Employment for Biomedical Technologists

Term	Academic Preparation	License/ Certification	Job Description	Employed by
Clinical Engineer	BS in life science or engineering; MS or Ph.D. in clinical engineering preferred	PE[a]+CCE	Manager of clinical engineering; interface between technology and health care personnel in clinical setting	Acute care hospitals, consulting services, medical equipment manufacturers (field application) or consultation
Biomedical Engineer (BME)	BS in life science or engineering; graduate study in biomedical engineering required (MS or Ph.D.)	None	Primarily research and teaching in biomedicine and biotechnology	Large corporations, research labs, and academic institutions
Medical Engineer (ME)	BS in engineering; MS or Ph.D. in biomedical or related specialty	None	Design and development of medical products and devices; some application and project engineering	Medical equipment manufacturers and medical laboratories or research labs
Biomedical Equipment Technician (BMET)	AAS in electrical technology or BS in electrical or biomedical technology	CBET[b]	Test, calibrate, maintain, and repair medical equipment and devices	Acute care hospitals, research labs, service organizations, medical equipment manufacturer

[a]PE only required for independent consulting.

[b]Not required if employed by a hospital.

Note: CBET = certified biomedical equipment technician; CCE = certified clinical engineer; PE = registered professional engineer.

- *Receiving adequate training:* Although the clinical engineering supervisor is trained to understand and maintain sophisticated equipment, his or her experience in personnel and financial management may be limited. As the director of a department, this individual should participate in training sessions, seminars, or academic programs that will strengthen his or her management background.
- *Establishing a risk management–based program:* Current standards of the Joint Commission on Accreditation of Healthcare Organizations provide flexibility in designing clinical equipment test programs. The department director needs to use that flexibility to ensure that the department's resources are being used effectively. For example, the director should schedule appropriate tests for critical care equipment to prevent patient harm due to improper operation.

☐ Organization and Staffing of the Department

The organization of the clinical engineering department is dependent upon the size (how much equipment will need to be tested and repaired) and mission of the hospital (long-term or acute care). Many clinical engineering departments evolved from plant operations or maintenance, and, as a result, are still within the organizational responsibility of that area.

Because the organization of clinical engineering departments varies from facility to facility, each department will be operated differently. However, there are some basic guidelines that will enable a department to be uniformly organized. These options are illustrated in figures 2-3 through 2-5.

Most small health care facilities (fewer than 150 beds) require the services of clinical engineering, but may not have sufficient resources or justification for a full-time, in-house biomedical technician. In many cases, a cost-effective solution is to contract with an outside agency that may be part of a large facility across town, a not-for-profit shared service "co-op," or a for-profit clinical engineering company. Outside service contracts can be less expensive if equipment test and repair needs are small. However, it is essential that the work be managed by the facility staff.

Figure 2-3. Clinical Engineering Department Staff Organization (Typical Small Hospital, 150 Beds)

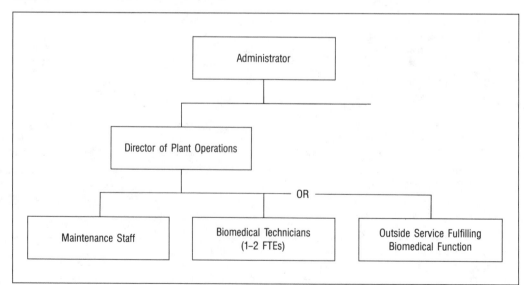

Figure 2-4. Clinical Engineering Department Staff Organization (Medium-Sized Community Hospital, 300 Beds)

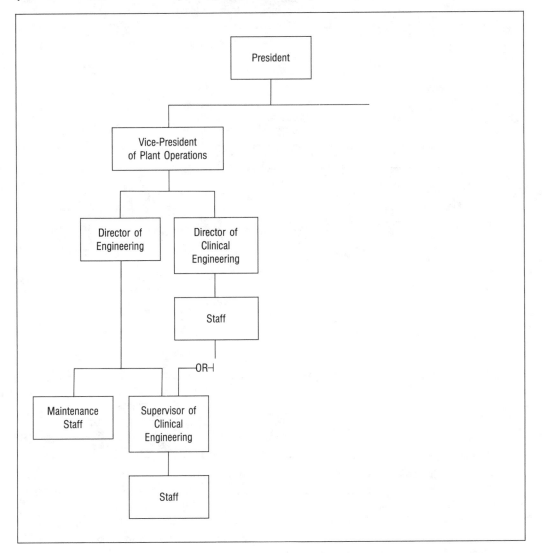

For small facilities, the biomedical engineering function (whether in-house or contract) normally reports to the director of maintenance, engineering, or plant operations. Because the primary responsibilities of clinical engineering in a small facility are to test and repair both patient and nonpatient equipment, day-to-day communication with the maintenance department is essential.

Communication, in fact, is important regardless of the facility's size. Because discussion with other staff members will routinely occur, especially with nursing and ancillary technician staff (those handling respiratory or physical therapy and so forth), these lines of communication must be supported by the clinical engineering department director.

In medium-sized facilities (approximately 300 beds), the clinical engineering department usually consists of a full-time staff of two to three biomedical technicians, with a supervisor or department director. Once again, the director of engineering is often charged with the responsibility to supervise clinical engineering. However, in some facilities, clinical engineering is a stand-alone department with a director who is linked directly to the vice-president of operations or the associate administrator. In some instances, the clinical engineering department may report to nursing, risk management, or even materials management.

**Figure 2-5. Clinical Engineering Department Staff Organization
(Large Community or University-Affiliated Medical Center, 500+ Beds)**

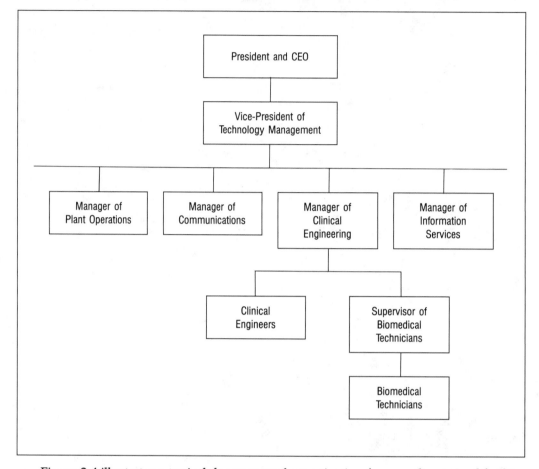

Figure 2-4 illustrates a typical departmental organization for a medium-sized facility. Most facilities of this size have clinical engineering departments staffed by biomedical technicians, but it is unusual for these facilities to hire a full-time clinical engineer. Because functions that require a certified clinical engineer (CCE) or a registered professional engineer (PE) may be necessary only several times per year, the facility may find it more cost-effective to retain a consulting clinical engineer. This individual can perform specific evaluations, conduct incident investigations, and undertake clinical engineering technical audits when needed.

Figure 2-5 illustrates a typical organizational chart for a large (more than 500 beds) urban health care facility or university-affiliated medical center. Because the effective management of technology in a large facility may require substantial expertise, it is not unusual to have managers or directors for plant operations, telecommunications, information services, and clinical engineering all reporting to a technology manager at the vice-presidential level.

Job Classifications

In health care facility clinical engineering departments, job titles, functions, and responsibilities vary significantly. However, there are generally four categories for biomedical technicians and two for clinical engineers. Figure 2-6 lists each of these categories in terms of generalized education, experience, supervision received, and supervision given. These descriptions are not intended to be all-encompassing, but do provide a sample framework for creating more specific job requirements and responsibilities.

Figure 2-6.   Summary of Clinical Engineering Department Job Descriptions

Title	Description	Qualifications	Supervision
BMET I	Junior, apprentice, or intern BMET; performs supervised tasks	AAS degree; no applicable experience	Closely supervised
BMET II	Biomedical technician working independently, doing equipment PM and repair of moderate difficulty	AAS degree; 2–3 years of applicable experience	Generally supervised
BMET III	Competently and independently performs skilled work of considerable difficulty	AAS or BSET degree; 5 or more years of applicable experience	May supervise other BMETs
BMET Supervisor	Performs independent work of significant complexity and coordinates and supervises others	AAS or BSET degree; certification and at least 5 years of applicable experience	Reports to department head; supervises other BMETs
Clinical Engineer	Provides training, analyzes systems, performs engineering consultation	BS or MS in clinical engineering, PE registration and CCE certification preferred	Supports BMETs and clinical personnel as necessary
Clinical Engineering Supervisor	Performs departmental planning and leadership; consults with other hospital department heads	BS or MS in clinical engineering; PE registration and CCE certification preferred; at least 5 years of applicable experience	Supervises and directs the clinical engineering department

Note: BMET = biomedical equipment technician; CCE = certified clinical engineer; PE = registered professional engineer; PM = preventive maintenance.

In-House or Outside Service Contracts

A dilemma often faced by a health care facility administrator is, "Should I create my own clinical engineering department, or hire an outside service company?" In addition to analyzing the cost, there are other considerations. For example, for a facility with fewer than 100 beds, it is usually less costly and more efficient to utilize a combination of outside service contractors and equipment manufacturer service representatives.

In most parts of the country, shared services have been organized through a consortium of facilities or as independent companies and are well equipped to test and repair most biomedical devices. Often, sophisticated laboratory and diagnostic radiology equipment is serviced by the manufacturer.

Facilities larger than 150 beds are usually able to justify at least one full-time biomedical technician for routine equipment tests and repairs. As with smaller facilities, it is prudent to complement this staff with service contracts when necessary. For facilities larger than 300 beds, or those institutions with specialty acute care services, it is usually cost-effective to staff a clinical engineering department with at least several full-time technicians and possibly a clinical engineer.

Although a well-managed in-house clinical engineering department is generally less costly than an outside service contract company, comparisons should be made on a cost-per-task basis rather than a dollars-per-hour basis. When outside service contracts begin to exceed 8 to 10 days per month, strong consideration should be given to employing a full-time, in-house technician.

In recent years, there has been much interest generated for maintenance insurance. The concept is that certain companies will offer a guaranteed fixed annual cost for the maintenance and repair of clinical equipment. Although this sounds attractive from a budget standpoint, total equipment maintenance and repair costs can be significantly less in the long term if equipment is well maintained and repairs are accomplished on a time-and-materials basis rather than a fixed-contract basis.

☐ Specific Tasks Done within the Department

When the first clinical engineering departments were started over 20 years ago, their primary function was to test and verify the safety of patient diagnostic and treatment devices and to keep them in operational condition. Although this remains a priority today, the typical department has many additional areas of responsibility that include the following:

- *Equipment safety testing:* Periodic tests are performed to determine whether equipment is safe to be used with patients. This particularly applies to electrical microshock and macroshock hazards. Completion of these tests is documented.
- *Equipment performance evaluation:* Equipment is routinely tested to verify that operation is within the original design parameters. An example would be the recording of the actual output of a defibrillator and checking it to see if the meter reading on the unit corresponds.
- *Equipment preventive maintenance:* Scheduled tasks are performed to extend the useful life of equipment, avoid unscheduled breakdowns, and minimize the need for repair. An example is lubrication of mechanical parts and replacement of power supply fan filters. Completion of these tasks is documented.
- *Equipment repair:* Whenever patient equipment fails to operate properly, the clinical engineering department is responsible for repairing the equipment. If the department is unable to complete the repair because of the equipment's complexity, a lack of replacement parts, or insufficient training or expertise, the department serves as a liaison to outside service representatives. In this role, the health care facility's biomedical technicians work with factory representatives to acquire additional equipment knowledge and verify the repair completion.
- *Equipment prepurchase evaluation:* Before clinical equipment purchases are made, a representative from the clinical engineering department provides consultation regarding equipment operation and serviceability. Frequently, the department performs sophisticated tests to verify proper operation and submits detailed reports to the equipment selection committee.
- *Postpurchase inspection* (often termed *incoming equipment evaluation*): When a device has been purchased, it is the responsibility of the clinical engineering department to certify that it is safe for use and that it performs within the required specifications. Documentation of the test results is provided to the user department as well as to the materials management staff.
- *In-service training:* Because there is such a wide variety of patient diagnostic and treatment equipment in the health care facility, it can be difficult to provide sufficient training for clinical and ancillary personnel. In this regard, the clinical engineering department can aid the nursing in-service department by conducting training sessions for equipment users.
- *Consultation with other departments:* Because the formal required training for clinical engineers and biomedical technicians includes courses in engineering principles, the clinical engineering staff can provide consultation to other departments within the facility. Examples include such diverse requests as equipment design modifications for research laboratories within the facility or helping with data analysis in the cardiovascular lab.
- *Product recalls:* Whenever medical products are recalled by the manufacturer, notification is sent to the health care facility. Often, the clinical engineering department is given the responsibility to review the nature of the recall, take action when necessary, report recommendations to the safety committee, and maintain a recall file for reference purposes.
- *Environmental testing:* As state and federal environmental requirements become more complex, the clinical engineering department can help to relieve the burden by

performing a wide variety of sound, light, and toxic gas tests. These can be especially cost-effective if the health care facility does not have a full-time staff industrial hygienist. Examples of tests include anesthesia waste gas, ethylene oxide, and laboratory formaldehyde gas level monitoring. The clinical engineering department may also work with the respiratory therapy and maintenance departments to provide evaluations of the medical gas vacuum systems.

- *Incident evaluations:* Whenever incidents that involve patient equipment occur in the facility, the clinical engineering department performs an equipment evaluation to identify and document equipment failures and user errors that have or may have an adverse effect on patient safety and/or the quality of care. This process is necessary to track trends of frequent failures, patient injuries, and so forth. There are various accreditation and legal requirements regarding incident evaluations.

- *Safety committee participation:* The clinical engineering department provides the safety committee with summaries that involve patient equipment failures, user errors, and reported equipment hazards to identify equipment performance and use problems. The summaries should be designed to provide relevant facts and classify the errors (for example, training, bed design, equipment age). When problems are identified, actions are taken to resolve them. Because of this requirement, the clinical engineering department should participate as a consultant to or member of the committee.

- *Service contract management:* In many facilities, the clinical engineering department is given the responsibility to coordinate all of the clinical equipment service contracts. Although this function has traditionally been fulfilled by materials management personnel or individual department heads, duplication of services can often be reduced by consolidating and coordinating contract management by the clinical engineering department.

- *Technology management:* Because of the proliferation of health care technology, many facilities are considering the addition of a *technology manager* or in some cases the creation of a technology services department. The responsibilities of this area include the review of technology equipment purchases, the management of technology maintenance, the control of technology contracts, and the monitoring of the impact of technology on the institution. All these functions could be provided by the clinical engineering department.

☐ Safety and Compliance

There are a few federal requirements that regulate the activities of clinical engineering departments within health care facilities, but for the most part it is voluntary organizations and accrediting bodies that define the organization, test criteria, and documentation standards for health care management.

Because many of these organizations are well known and promulgate recommended standards that are widely followed, some state and local agencies have adopted their publications as legally enforceable. The following section briefly describes some of these organizations.

Government Organizations

Several U.S. government agencies have been organized to regulate health devices. Following are some of those agencies that apply to clinical engineering:

- Within the federal Food and Drug Administration (FDA), the Center for Devices and Radiological Health (CDRH) regulates several areas formerly handled by the Bureau of Medical Devices and the Bureau for Radiological Health. The CDRH regulates diagnostic product standards and the development of new products and is responsible for ensuring that products emitting radiation from lasers, ultrasound, and X-ray equipment comply with standards specified by the Radiation and Control for Health and Safety Act—PL.9602.

- The Occupational Safety and Health Administration (OSHA) regulates working conditions for all health care employees, whereas the National Institute for Occupational Safety and Health (NIOSH) serves as a research arm for OSHA. The NIOSH does not have any regulatory authority.
- The Federal Communications Commission (FCC) controls devices that emit energy in the radio frequency range. This includes ultrasound, diathermy, X-ray, computer, and communications equipment.
- The National Bureau of Standards (NBS) provides reference calibration standards for medical instruments.
- The Veterans Administration (VA) creates its own test standards to use within the VA system. These specifications may be adopted by non-VA hospitals, but on a purely voluntary basis.

International Organizations

The International Electrical Commission (IEC) and the International Organization for Standards (IOS) provide standards for use worldwide, and their influence is expected to increase when the European community removes additional trade barriers in 1992.

National Voluntary Standards Organizations

The primary organizations concerned with voluntary medical device standards include the American Society for Testing and Materials (ASTM), the Association for the Advancement of Medical Instrumentation (AAMI), the National Fire Protection Association (NFPA), and Underwriters Laboratories (UL). In some areas, the adoption of NFPA and UL standards by local, regional, and state authorities requires compliance under penalty of law. Some of the standards that have been adopted by regulatory agencies that affect clinical engineering departments include:

- NFPA 70, 1990, Article 517 of the National Electrical Code, "Health Care Facilities"
- NFPA 99, 1990, chapter 7 of Health Care Facilities, "Electrical Equipment"
- UL 544, 1988, "Electrical Medical and Dental Equipment"

Accreditation Organizations

Of major interest to most health care facilities is the Joint Commission on Accreditation of Healthcare Organizations (Joint Commission), which accredits participating health care facilities through an on-site survey process. The survey includes specific questions related to equipment management. Although limited flexibility is permitted in meeting the standards, the following characteristics are required in its 1991 *Accreditation Manual for Hospitals:*

1. Written criteria must be established to determine which equipment will be included on a control inventory.
2. Equipment that is included on the inventory list must be tested at specified intervals, and the results of these tests must be documented.
3. Training must be provided to those who use and maintain the equipment.
4. The program must identify and document certain equipment failures and user errors.
5. When applicable, summaries of these failures and errors must be reported to at least one of the following for evaluation, action, and resolution: safety officer, quality assurance, or risk management.

☐ Program Evaluation

As with any department, clinical engineering is charged with the responsibility for developing a process that measures the success or failure of its program. The clinical engineering department uses both quality control as well as quality assurance (QA) techniques to measure its performance.

Quality control methods are used to verify whether certain measurable quantities are maintained within a defined range. Examples include determining whether equipment preventive maintenance tasks are performed within scheduled times and according to prescribed procedures. Also, repairs that require recalls (indicating questionable repair quality) may be tracked, or the number of equipment user errors as a percentage of unscheduled work orders can be documented. Each of these examples includes measuring a result and comparing it with a preexisting set of standards.

On the other hand, quality assurance is more difficult to determine. To have indicators by which to measure, the department needs to develop a mission statement that has built-in measures. This will allow the department to readily measure its job performance through a review and evaluation process.

A process that can be useful in developing a QA program might include the following steps:

1. Determine measurable parameters that will serve as indicators to the level of quality that is desired; for example, the percentage of preventive maintenance (PM) tasks that are completed according to schedule.
2. Collect data to determine a current level of compliance with the parameters listed in (1) above; for example, document the PM completion percentage each month for at least three months.
3. Set desirable targets and thresholds to define *minimum acceptable* and *maximum achievable* levels; for example, a minimum acceptable on-time PM completion rate might be 75 percent, whereas a maximal achievable level would be 100 percent.
4. Create strategies to ensure acceptable levels while attempting to attain the maximally achievable ones; for example, develop a PM priority system and/or redesign PM procedures to reflect a risk-based approach. For the long term, analyze staffing productivity to determine the need for the staff changes.
5. Take necessary action and monitor the resulting changes; for example, establish PM priorities and determine the effect on PM completion rate.
6. Continue to monitor the parameters, take appropriate action, and redefine the thresholds as necessary; for example, use of the risk-based approach to PM procedures can reduce the average PM time and thereby increase the on-time PM completion percentage from 75 percent to 85 percent.

The measurement of quality control parameters with accompanying indicators depends on the needs of each health care facility. Example parameters that may be used to develop a quality control program are listed in figure 2-7.

☐ Summary

The formation of the clinical engineering department within the health care facility has resulted from the need to effectively manage the rapidly increasing field of diagnostic and treatment devices and equipment. The typical clinical engineering department is staffed by biomedical technicians and, in large facilities, clinical engineers who test and maintain the clinical equipment. Often, the staff provides other functions such as pre-purchase evaluation, special consultation, environmental testing, and in-service training. Although the clinical engineering department usually reports to the engineering and

Figure 2-7. Typical Quality Control Measurements for Clinical Engineering Departments

Indicator	Measurement Quality	Minimum Acceptable Threshold	Maximum Acceptable Threshold
On-time PM completion	Percentage	75%	100%
Ultimate PM completion	Percentage	90%	100%
Average equipment repair time	Hours	1.5 hours	1.0 hours
Repair/recall rate within 48 hours	Percentage	5%	0%
Staff productivity	Percentage	70%	100%
Average equipment failure rate	Mean Time Between Failure	>PM interval	No failure
User error rate	Percentage of unscheduled work orders	25%	0%
Departmental budget	Percentage of expense compared to budget	100% of budget	Variable
Questionnaire results	Qualitative rating 1–10	8.0	10.0

Note: PM = preventive maintenance.

maintenance body within the health care facility, the staff needs to communicate with the nursing, risk management, and administrative departments.

Management of the clinical engineering department should include the establishment of a separate cost center to permit financial responsibility. Adequate staffing and resources should be provided so that a risk management–based program can be created. In addition, specific quality control indicators should be adopted so that program effectiveness can be evaluated and documented. The codes and standards that regulate clinical equipment tests that are performed by the clinical engineering department include government, international, and national voluntary standards organizations, as well as accreditation organizations.

□ References and Bibliography

Emergency Care Research Institute. Technology management: preparing your hospital for the 1990s. *Health Technology* 3(1), Spring 1980.

Joint Commission on Accreditation of Healthcare Organizations. *Accreditation Manual for Hospitals, 1991 edition.* Oakbrook Terrace, IL: JCAHO, 1991.

Keil, O. R. The challenge of building quality into clinical engineering programs. In: *Plant, Technology, and Safety Management: Translating Theory into Practice.* Chicago: Joint Commission on Accreditation of Healthcare Organizations (series), 1990.

McBride, S., Glidden, T., and Riesebey, R. L. *The Guide to Biomedical Standards.* 15th ed. Brea, CA: Quest Publishing Co., 1988–89.

Nader, R. Ralph Nader's most shocking exposé. *Ladies' Home Journal*, Mar. 1971, pp. 98–179.

National Fire Protection Association. *NFPA 70: National Electrical Code, 1990.* Quincy, MA: NFPA, 1990.

National Fire Protection Association. *NFPA 99: Health Care Facilities Standard, 1987 edition.* Quincy, MA: NFPA, 1987.

Newhouse, V. L., Bell, D.S., Tackel, I.S., and others. The future of clinical engineering in the 1990s. *Journal of Clinical Engineering* 14(5):417–30, Sept.–Oct. 1989.

Pacela, A. F. 1989 survey of hospital salaries and job responsibilities for clinical engineers and biomedical technicians. *Journal of Clinical Engineering* 14(4):313–29, July–Aug. 1989.

Slack, G. D. Personal data base, 1991.

Slack, G. D., and McKinney, J. W. *Training Manual for Biomedical Equipment Technicians, Part I.* Chicago: American Society for Hospital Engineering, 1989.

Walter, C. W. *Electrical Hazards in Hospitals: Proceedings of a Workshop.* Washington, DC: National Academy of Sciences, 1970, p. 60.

Webster, J. G., and Cork, A. M.. *Clinical Engineering Principles and Practices.* Englewood Cliffs, NJ: Prentice-Hall, 1979.

Chapter 3
Environmental Services

Aralee Scardina

☐ Overview

The most common term used to describe the department responsible for the cleaning and general appearance of a health care facility is *environmental services*. However, this multifaceted department may be known by many different names, including housekeeping services, facility management, domestic services, institutional services, or janitorial services.

The value of an environmental services department is immediately evident to everyone who enters the health care facility. The work of this department can create a strong initial impression about the cleanliness of the overall operation and the services the facility provides.

A well-maintained health care facility also has a definite positive effect on the people working there. A clean workplace makes everyone's job easier and more pleasant.

People who work in the environmental services department come from diverse backgrounds and generally can be trained to do this work in a relatively short period of time. This department offers employment opportunities not only for individuals reentering the work force after many years of not working outside the home, but also for those who have limited skills, restricted physical abilities, or are new to this country. Students needing flexible hours also can benefit from the opportunities offered by this department.

In addition to having responsibility for cleaning the health care facility, the environmental services department has a number of other duties that can include grounds keeping, minor maintenance, pest control, and waste management. These and other departmental duties are discussed in this chapter.

☐ Department Head Responsibilities

The environmental services department is usually headed by a manager who is involved in the day-to-day operation of the department. His or her principal responsibilities include approving scheduling, formulating departmental policy and budget, and helping train employees.

The position calls for prior training and/or experience in housekeeping procedures and the management of people. Important skills include knowledge of work analysis, measurement, and distribution. Environmental services managers must also be able to effectively communicate orally and in writing. Because the sanitation of the hospital environment is so important, one of the manager's primary responsibilities is developing employee skills and motivating employees to use them.

Guest Relations

Managers of environmental services departments have several responsibilities in the area of guest relations. Because environmental services workers have a great deal of patient contact, it is important that they present a positive, professional image. An impression of all hospital personnel is often formed by patient and visitor contact with environmental services workers. Managers should ensure that environmental services staff wear clean, well-pressed, and appropriate uniforms and that their equipment is clean, operable, and in good condition.

Satisfaction with the physical environment also influences the patient's overall opinion of the facility. Therefore, a system should be designed and implemented to aggressively seek out the patient's level of satisfaction. Face-to-face interviews with patients will give the environmental services manager invaluable information about the services the department provides, as well as ideas that can improve the way the department's services are delivered.

A simple interview form (figure 3-1) can produce valuable insight into the patient's response to the services he or she receives. An added benefit to this type of patient interaction is information that can be passed on to other departments that will help them improve the quality of the services they provide, as well.

Employee Relations

In addition to maintaining guest relations, environmental services managers must communicate effectively with departmental staff members. Good employee relations and communication are crucial to the success of employee performance. Providing a clean environment requires teamwork, and teamwork is based on friendly and productive interaction among employees. Key to effective communication is ensuring that employees understand their supervisors' expectations.

Although most personnel evaluation systems are designed to provide an annual performance review, there should be a system for letting environmental services employees know whether they are meeting expectations throughout the year. This system could be as informal as offering a word of encouragement or as detailed as designing a work incentive program that recognizes an employee for a job well done.

□ Organization of the Department and Staffing

The organization of the environmental services department can vary a great deal with the size of the facility. The basic structure will usually consist of a department head, managers, supervisors and/or work leaders, a training position (either a specific position or a dual position of supervisor and/or work leader), and a working staff responsible for the day-to-day tasks.

The working staff may be organized on several different levels depending on the skills required and the responsibilities. A fairly common practice is to separate workers into two groups: one that carries out the routine daily cleaning tasks, and one that is trained to operate the power machinery. Organizational examples of a housekeeping department and a larger environmental services department are shown in figures 3-2 and 3-3.

Figure 3-1. Housekeeping Services Patient Satisfaction Interview Form

Room #: _____

Date: _____

Patient Name: _____

Cleanliness	Satisfactory	Unsatisfactory
Room	_____	_____
Bathrooms	_____	_____
Carpet	_____	_____
Floors	_____	_____
Walls	_____	_____
Windows	_____	_____

Housekeeping Staff		
Response to requests	_____	_____
Courtesy	_____	_____
Appearance	_____	_____

Comfort		
Bed	_____	_____
Furniture	_____	_____
Decor	_____	_____

	Very Satisfactory	Satisfactory	Unsatisfactory
Overall Satisfaction	_____	_____	_____

Comments: _____

_____

_____

Figure 3-2. Housekeeping Services Organizational Chart

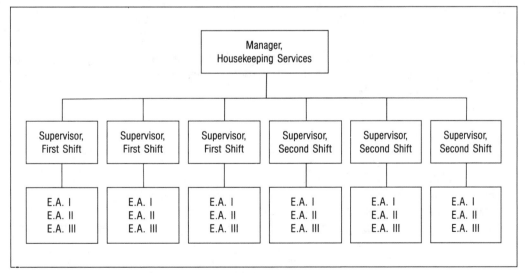

Note: There are three teams for each shift, and each team works in a different area of the facility.

E.A. = environmental assistant.

31

Figure 3-3. A Medical Center Environmental Services Department Organizational Chart

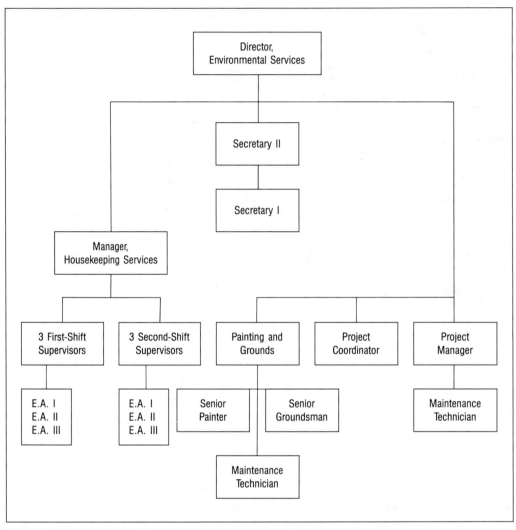

Note: E.A. = environmental assistant.

As the administration weighs the cost of daily operations, it must determine how to provide the most effective and efficient services. There are two options: in-house services and contract services.

In-House Services

With in-house services, the employees hired to clean and the procedures they use remain under the control of the organization's administration. To assure quality standards, training programs tailored to fit the facility's needs should be designed.

An in-house department also offers the flexibility of making adjustments to meet the demands of the changing health care field without the need for costly negotiations. Other advantages offered by an in-house service include:

- *Loyalty:* Because an in-house department has no outside influence, its leadership has one loyalty—the health care facility.

- *Cost:* Because an in-house department is not established as an organized profit center, its operation is usually less expensive.
- *Leadership:* The leadership of an in-house department can be trained and motivated to fulfill the expectations of the administration.

Contract Services

If the facility's needs cannot be met by an in-house department, the option is to contract outside services. For instance, an outside service may be able to take a very troubled environmental services department and provide effective trouble-shooting and program planning. It could also be helpful in a catastrophic situation such as a flood, a fire, or a construction cleanup where an in-house service needs assistance.

The cost and service comparisons of an outside versus an inside service must be carefully considered before a commitment is made. The facility as well as the contractor must understand and be able to meet each other's expectations. If comprehensive performance standards are not established before the contractor begins service, the administration may find that many less-obvious tasks (which had been routinely completed by the in-house department) are no longer being done because they were not specified in the contract with the outside service. Thus the lower cost may not be a bargain if expected services are not performed.

Another consideration is the status of equipment. Often a contractor's bid will include the replacement of all equipment as it becomes necessary. It is important that any decision regarding contracted services clearly define ownership of equipment.

It is likewise important to recognize that if the contracted company retains ownership of the equipment, all the equipment leaves if the contract is terminated. The replacement cost of all the equipment at one time could place an organization in a no-choice situation. Because replacing all the environmental services equipment would be costly, it might be necessary to continue the contract service whether the institution wants to or not.

☐ Specific Tasks Done within the Department

The environmental services department's responsibilities include cleaning, some tasks formerly done by nurses, grounds keeping, painting services, property management, assets and equipment disposal, signage, minor maintenance, pest control, waste management, and recycling.

Cleaning

The largest single task of an environmental services department is cleaning the facility. This includes all environmental surfaces (the tops, bottoms, outsides, and insides of all furniture and walls, doors, floors, sinks, showers, tubs, toilets, and so forth) that can be cleaned with a germicide rather than sterilized or do not require a specialized cleaning procedure. Technical or medical equipment is not included.

Occasionally, a question arises regarding which department should clean a specific item. In the past, medical equipment was less sophisticated and could usually be cleaned by the environmental services staff. However, because today's equipment often requires persons specially trained to clean it properly, the cleaning task would be inappropriate for environmental services workers to perform. A good rule of thumb is that, if the equipment has knobs, buttons, or dials that could be moved in the process of cleaning—and such movement could affect the equipment's operation or results—cleaning should be done by a technician rather than an environmental services worker. This reduces the possibility of a piece of equipment working improperly because its settings were disturbed.

Other duties carried out by the environmental services worker include cleaning and replacing window coverings, transporting soiled linen, and removing trash.

Tasks Formerly Done by Nurses

Environmental services workers can also perform duties that will free medical personnel for more direct patient care. Some of these tasks include making beds, straightening bed linens for patients, passing water pitchers, or performing any cleaning functions being done by nursing personnel.

By accepting nonpatient care duties previously assigned to the nursing staff, the environmental services department can become an even more valuable asset to the facility. The value of this kind of service can be seen when nursing positions are used exclusively for direct patient care, which enables nurses to provide care more efficiently. By assuming the role of providing nonpatient care duties, environmental services establishes itself as responsive and involved in an overall service-oriented organization.

Before the department assumes these roles, however, permission must be channeled through proper administrative routes. The duties being considered for reassignment should be appropriate for the environmental services department.

Grounds Keeping

This function involves the landscaping, planting, pruning, trimming, watering, and fertilizing of shrubs, trees, and grass. Grounds workers are usually responsible for snow removal and ice control as well. Often the grounds workers will move boxes, equipment, furniture, set up rooms for meetings and conferences, and help start cars in cold weather.

Painting Services

Painting services is responsible for maintaining fresh paint on walls and other surfaces. Other duties may include refinishing furniture, repainting metal equipment, repairing plaster, hanging wallpaper, and refinishing doors and other wooden surfaces. This function may also involve hanging pictures, drapery rods, and blinds, and performing minor repairs on wall-mounted furnishings.

Property Management

Often health care facilities acquire houses, commercial buildings, and other properties around the institution for future expansion. These buildings are often used as housing for medical residents or students, as guest houses for out-of-town relatives of patients, or as office space for the hospital. They also are rented to the general public as a source of revenue.

Environmental services often maintains and provides cleaning services for these buildings as well, in which case a property coordinator works out of the environmental services department. The property coordinator prepares and maintains tenant leases, whether the tenants are private citizens or hospital employees. This position is also responsible for coordinating routine and special repairs to the properties and cleaning upon turnover of tenants. Moreover, the property coordinator serves as a liaison between surrounding neighbors and the health care facility.

Assets and Equipment Disposal

When a piece of equipment is replaced by the medical facility, it is often the environmental services department's responsibility to move out the old equipment and move in the new equipment. The department would then handle the disposal of replaced equipment.

The orderly disposal of hospital assets is a vital function for any organization. Space is an expensive commodity, and a facility cannot afford to dedicate any of its space to house unused equipment. This equipment can also represent a source of revenue for the institution because there is a ready market for it. For example, veterinarians often purchase old medical equipment.

Equipment that is too old or no longer serves an institution's purpose is often welcomed by small clinics and private practitioners. Old office and patient furnishings are very salable items. Some health care institutions have regular rummage sales and invite their employees and the general public to purchase equipment and furniture that are no longer used.

Moreover, if all avenues of sale are exhausted, discarded equipment and furniture can often be donated to organizations either in the community or in emerging and third-world nations.

Signage

People are often overwhelmed when they walk through the door of a health care facility. They must find a specific place, no matter how large or small the building. One way to eliminate unnecessary confusion is the proper placement of signage. Because environmental services workers work throughout the facility, they are very aware of the kinds of signage that will facilitate the movement of patients and visitors.

The environmental services department can also ensure that signs are well placed, easy to read, and clearly direct people to the various departments, floors, and wings of the facility. Traveling through a facility can be easier if a good signage program is in place, and it could prove to be an exceptionally good guest relations tool.

New technology in sign making has made it possible for inexperienced people to make very professional, permanent signs. The environmental services department can also coordinate any outside signage contracts.

Minor Maintenance

Minor repairs requiring "handyman" skills are often part of the tasks performed by an environmental services department. Some of the minor maintenance tasks delegated to this department are faucet repair, drain cleaning, drapery rod and window blinds repair, light bulb changing, and air conditioner/air filter cleaning. Simple repairs on housekeeping equipment are also done by this department.

Pest Control

From time to time, even the most well-kept institution will have a problem with pests. Often, roaches, fleas, and lice will come in with a patient's belongings. It is extremely important to stop the spread of these very prolific pests as soon as possible, and this can be done safely by spraying patient areas.

Certain areas (receiving, food storage, and so forth) require a regular spraying program. This is usually accomplished with a contract pest control service.

From time to time, rodents can become a problem, especially when the weather turns cold. Sometimes, even larger animals such as raccoons, opossums, and rats can invade a facility. With larger animals, it is better to call a pest control company. The environmental services worker can set a mousetrap and empty it, but larger animals need to be handled by a pest control professional.

Waste Management

The handling of waste from a medical facility has taken on a new twist in recent years. Because of public perception and government reaction, health care–generated waste is separated into several categories. In some states, *all* medical trash is treated as if it poses a hazard to the general public.

A critical factor in waste disposal is the system set up inside the building to separate, store, and dispose of the various types of trash. Several federal agencies (EPA, OSHA, the Department of Transportation, and others) impose specific regulations. In addition, waste-handling requirements may differ from state to state.

There are several trash streams that must be managed within the health care facility. They are:

- *Solid waste:* This includes paper, kitchen garbage, office trash, and noncontaminated trash from patient areas.
- *Medical, infectious, or potentially infectious waste:* This includes needles, sharps, and trash from treatment areas or isolation patient rooms.
- *Chemotherapy waste:* This includes trash consisting of IV bags, tubing, gloves, disposable gowns, and so forth from the chemotherapy treatment of cancer patients.
- *Radioactive waste:* This consists of materials used to diagnose and treat patients with special requirements. This waste could include syringes, tubing, gloves, masks, gowns worn by the care giver, and other patient care items. It could also include trash from the room occupied by a patient of a radiation implant treatment as well as low-level radioactive laboratory waste.
- *Hazardous waste:* This is usually chemical, as covered by the Resource Conservation and Recovery Act, and requires very special handling and disposal.

Solid waste is usually eligible for placement in landfill facilities. Medical, infectious, or potentially infectious material must be clearly marked from the time it enters the trash stream until it is destroyed. Every person coming in contact with this material must be aware of the potential for infection. Furthermore, the laws of each state must be studied and understood to be sure medical waste is being properly handled. Therefore, all departments need to know the proper methods of disposal for all items they handle.

Chemotherapy waste must be placed in clearly labeled, separate containers. The materials used in chemotherapy are toxic and must be handled in a way that ensures the safety of all who come in contact with them. To be rendered harmless, chemotherapy waste must be incinerated at regulated temperatures.

If the medical or chemotherapy waste is disposed of off-site to be incinerated, a comprehensive tracking system is required. Commonly referred to as a manifest system, this system is required by many states and is a prudent practice for any health care facility. However, there are some alternate methods to medical waste disposal, such as sterilization, encapsulation, and grinding with disinfectants. It is important to look at all methods to determine which is most workable and cost-effective for each particular health care facility.

Briefly described, sterilization is a process that renders the infectious properties of the waste harmless through steam, ethylene oxide gas, or chemical (a disinfectant) sterilization. If the amount of waste is small, such as one or two bags, most health care facilities have autoclaves or gas sterilizers that can handle the task. Most hospitals, however, would need to invest in a cart-sized sterilizer to take care of a larger volume. The primary disadvantage of this system is that many landfill sites are opposed to accepting sterilized infectious waste.

The encapsulation method is used primarily for the disposal of sharps. Machinery collects the infectious material in a bin. Next, plastic material is added as heat and pressure are applied, tightly sealing the infectious waste in a solid plastic cylinder. Because this technology is relatively new, little is known about the acceptance of this method by landfill companies.

Another fairly new technology is a machine that grinds the waste while mixing it with a disinfectant. This process reduces the volume of the waste and destroys its appearance, which can make the waste more acceptable for landfill disposal.

The waste from a patient being treated with radioactive materials should be separate and handled only by a person trained in radiation safety. In addition, this disposal method requires knowledge of Nuclear Regulatory Commission codes and those of other regulating bodies.

Hazardous waste requires very special handling and disposal. The most common hazardous waste found in hospitals is from the laboratory (xylene and reagent chemicals) and the radiology department (used developing solution). A considerable investment in specialized equipment will enable the facility to recycle chemicals on-site. This process leaves a smaller amount of waste, which still requires special handling.

Very few health care organizations can handle disposal of these items on-site. A complete list of those substances requiring this very specialized disposal can be found in the Resource Conservation and Recovery Act. The best resource for the disposal of these items is an experienced hazardous waste disposal company.

Recycling

The entire issue of disposable materials has come under very close scrutiny. A hospital can encourage recycling and energy conservation among its departments by implementing comprehensive programs, including waste-handling task forces.

The disposable items used in environmental services are few when compared to the many disposables used throughout a health care facility. Even so, the facilitywide number of disposables has, predictably, created a sizable waste problem. Environmental services departments often participate in recycling projects and conservation efforts through coordinating projects and collecting and storing materials. In addition, if the facility is recycling aluminum cans, housekeeping staff may help separate cans from other refuse and haul them to a general collection location. With diminishing landfill sites, tougher clean air standards, and the drain of natural resources, it is difficult to justify the use of throwaway products.

Many institutions are already recycling office paper. At first, recycling was done to preserve forests, but now it is being encouraged to reduce the amount of waste that must be disposed of by a health care facility.

Some state legislatures are enacting laws that will require disposable items to be recycled. For instance, the 1989 Wisconsin Act 335 lists materials found in health care institutions that can be recycled. Under this legislation, health care facilities are not permitted to place recyclable materials in landfill sites.

The list of materials that can be recycled is growing almost daily. Office paper is an example of a product that can be recycled. Other items include aluminum cans, aluminum scrap, corrugated paper, newsprint, plastics such as jugs, bottles and containers, glass, Styrofoam, and metal cans.

Aside from the obvious reduction in hauling costs and landfill fees by removing these items from the trash system, revenue can be realized from recycling these materials. Such items as high-grade office and computer paper or aluminum offer consistent financial returns to the organization. Although other materials may not yield high returns, they will offset the cost of hauling and will stay out of the trash compactor and the landfills.

☐ Equipment and Technology

An efficiently operated environmental services department will have equipment and supplies that are suited to completing assigned tasks. Basic pieces of equipment required for general cleaning are pails, mops, buckets, wringers, trash and linen carts, general cleaning carts, dust mops, brooms, dustpans, and vacuum cleaners.

For floor care, additional equipment such as single-disc scrubbers and wet pickups is required. A wide range of choice is available for carpet care. Machinery is available.

that will dry-clean the carpet, extract dampness, or use dry foam in the cleaning process. It is important to match the system to the recommendations of the carpet manufacturer.

Automatic housekeeping equipment can be very helpful. Although automatic equipment may have a high price tag, the cost may be offset by savings in labor. For example, it is less expensive to clean a corridor with an automatic scrubber than to mop it by hand. It is less costly to spray-paint a piece of furniture than to paint it by hand.

Any automated process usually results in a labor savings. However, time studies, demonstrations, contacts with others in the profession, and any other information available should be studied before making costly and possibly unnecessary purchases.

In addition to equipment, there are some basic supplies required. The most important supply is an infection control–approved germicide, which is used for the routine cleaning of all environmental surfaces. Also needed are various cleaning products for other surfaces such as glass, metal, wood, porcelain, and a host of different wall coverings.

Because a number of products can be used for several purposes, one very important aspect of choosing supplies is versatility. To ensure that products are used in a cost-efficient manner, it is necessary to have ample products on hand and require that each product be used properly. The efficient use of supplies will result in substantial cost savings to the department.

One of the greatest challenges facing the leadership of an environmental services department is ensuring that equipment is kept in good working order. From broken wringer springs to worn-down casters, the care of equipment is a singularly frustrating and never-ending task. A high-quality maintenance program for equipment begins with the employees who work with it. A training program, formal inspections (figure 3-4), and procedures that clearly outline the process and its expectations must be in place to assist employees and supervisors in keeping the equipment in top condition.

In recent years, the use of disposable goods such as mops, cleaning cloths, dust mops, and dust cloths has increased. Although an attractive option may be to have clean equipment on hand, the impact of these disposable items on the trash stream has caused many users to question their value. Although there is little doubt that there is a place for disposables in the environmental services department, the benefits must be carefully weighed against all costs.

One very important factor to consider is that most disposables are made, in some part, of paper, which is a source of dust and lint. With the increased use of disposable cleaning and linen items, many health care organizations have noticed that the level of dust and lint within the building is higher.

□ Safety and Compliance

Many regulatory agencies, voluntary organizations, and accrediting bodies have jurisdiction throughout sections of a health care organization, and the environmental services department is no exception. Following are agencies that have an impact on environmental services.

Joint Commission on Accreditation of Healthcare Organizations

The majority of specific requirements for the environmental services department can be found in the Infection Control section of the Joint Commission's *Accreditation Manual for Hospitals*. The responsibilities of the environmental services director can be found under the heading of Housekeeping Services in the index of the manual. These responsibilities include development of procedures and schedules; training and supervision of personnel; use, cleaning, and care of equipment; liaison with the infection control committee; and documentation of all of the above.

Figure 3-4. Housekeeping Department Equipment Inspection Quality Control Form

St. Luke's Hospital
Milwaukee, Wisconsin
Environmental Services Dept.

HOUSEKEEPING DEPARTMENT
EQUIPMENT INSPECTION QUALITY CONTROL
X-2496 4/84

EMPLOYEE/AREA			TIME	DATE

PERCENTAGE STANDARD _____ %   INSPECTED BY _____

MACHINE ☐ OPERATIONAL ☐ NON-OPERATIONAL ☐ NEEDS REPAIR-SEE COPY ON MACHINE

ELEMENTS	S	U	ELEMENTS	S	U
EXTRACTOR			(WET DRY VAC con't.)		
Solution Tank			Hose		
Recovery Tank & Filter			Squeegee		
Cords			Wand		
Hoses			Exterior		
Wheels			Battery		
Exterior					
Wands			VACUUM		
Upholstery Wand			Bag		
			Bag Housing		
HOST MACHINES			Exterior		
Exterior			Wheels		
Brushes			Brushes		
Hood-Inside			Underside		
Carrier			Cord-Hoses		
Cord					
			AUTO SCRUBBER		
CIMEX MACHINES			Solution Tank		
Tank			Recovery Tank		
Exterior			Filter		
Wheels			Tires		
Brushes			Battery		
Cord			Exterior		
			Squeegee		
SCRUBBER			Drive Plates		
Tank					
Exterior			WHIRLAMATIC		
Wheels			Exterior		
Cord			Hood		
Drive Plate			Wheels		
			Battery		
WRINGER			Motor Compartment		
Handle					
Inside			SWEEPER		
Outside			Filter		
			Exterior		
WET DRY VAC			Collection Bin		
Tank			Wheels		
Hood			Battery		
Wheels			Underside & Inside Frame		
Cord					

RECORD COMMENTS HERE - CONTINUE ON REVERSE SIDE IF NECESSARY

_____

_____

_____

_____

_____

Employee/s Initials _____

Source: Reprinted, with permission, from Saint Luke's Medical Center, Milwaukee.

The prime objective of the department is to provide a hygienic environment for patients and staff. It is important for the environmental services director to become very familiar with the Joint Commission manual and the references to housekeeping practices that are mentioned in many of the individual department chapters.

In the event of a fire or mass casualty, the Joint Commission requires that environmental services workers know what to do, whom they report to, and where to go. Other areas of awareness are worker safety, equipment safety, and hazardous materials management. A program of safe working practices must also be established and monitored within the department.

Occupational Safety and Health Administration

The nature of the work in environmental services requires employees to be well trained in safety hazards that could put them at risk. The importance of the role of environmental services employees should be strongly emphasized. As a result, the Occupational Safety and Health Administration (OSHA) has issued numerous regulations that affect environmental services employees. For example, there are OSHA rules covering the use of ladders, electrical safety, and lifting techniques.

The Occupational Safety and Health Administration defines a hazardous chemical or product as follows: ". . . one is considered hazardous if it has been determined to be carcinogenic, corrosive, skin or eye irritating, likely to cause an allergic reaction, toxic or dangerous to certain bodily organs." The possible dangers, their precautions, and their treatment are detailed in the material safety data sheet (MSDS) for each product. The MSDS must be provided by the supplier of the product.

There are various exposure hazards from the many different cleaning products; some of the dangers may be to skin, others are to the eyes or respiratory system. Employees must know the physical and health hazards of chemicals and the protective measures to take to prevent injury. For example, most chemicals used in routine cleaning tasks require special precautions to prevent exposure or injury to the environmental services worker.

Guidelines have also been set on an employee's right to know about other substances and materials that he or she comes in contact with on the job. Because environmental services workers routinely handle soiled linen and trash, they must be informed of the possible dangers of these items. For example, linen may come from a patient who has a contagious disease. Because it may not be properly identified as being contaminated, all soiled linen must be handled as if it were infectious. Workers also should understand that the trash they handle may have harmful material in it.

To meet OSHA regulations outlined in the Hazard Communication Standard, procedures outlining those dangers and the safety practices that must be taken by employees must be followed. Moreover, protective clothing and equipment must be provided to workers to ensure that they do not come in contact with hazardous chemicals. This could include personal protective equipment such as coveralls, appropriate gloves, safety glasses, or other face protection.

The possibility of inspections, citations, and fines accompanies any regulation or standard. The Occupational Safety and Health Administration inspects facilities to determine whether the interest of the Hazard Communication Standard is being carried out. The primary reason for inspections is to ensure that the safety and health of employees are protected from the dangerous effects of hazardous chemicals. If environmental services directors ensure that their safety programs meet the Hazard Communication Standard requirements, the possibility of employee complaints and injuries that result in inspections will be reduced.

U.S. Environmental Protection Agency

Legislation and guidance governing the handling and disposal of medical waste and hazardous materials are developed by the U.S. Environmental Protection Agency (EPA).

This federal agency defines and regulates the flow of hazardous/medical waste, establishes requirements for facilities to develop tracking programs, and outlines systems for dealing with environmental accidents such as leaks and spills.

☐ Program Evaluation

To ensure that the environmental services department is running smoothly, procedures must be in place to prevent the spread of germs and establish operating standards for the department.

Infection Control

One of the main objectives of the environmental services department is to ensure that the building remains as germfree as possible. This applies to routine cleaning as well as special cases where a patient's illness is infectious enough to be a potential danger to others.

Step-by-step procedures must be prepared to ensure that all environmental surfaces are cleaned on a routine basis and that cleaning standards are met. It is essential that environmental services workers have a written procedure for every task they are to perform. These guidelines explain precisely what the workers are to do, how they are to do it, the order for performing each step, the equipment and supplies they will need, and approximately how long it will take them to do the task. To be effective, procedures must be reviewed and revised regularly. Figure 3-5 is an example of a step-by-step procedure.

The next step is an effective training program that is to be taken by each environmental services worker. Many times, training is conducted using the buddy system, where good workers take new employees along with them to watch and imitate their performance.

The buddy system is better than nothing—but not much better. The problem is that mistakes or unauthorized methods and variations can be perpetuated that may lead to difficulties in performance. An experienced trainer using a competency-based training program provides an environmental services department with a staff that is consistent, professional, and effective.

Every organization has some employees who perform at above-average levels or show a tendency toward leadership. They have good verbal and written skills and a good understanding of departmental goals. Taking the time to teach these employees how to train can be cost-effective in meeting those goals.

Using a training checklist (figure 3-6) that outlines a comprehensive training process provides the trainer with a mechanism that documents specific training activities. This kind of training program also encourages a career path for future environmental services leaders.

To avoid unnecessary employee exposure to certain illnesses, the Centers for Disease Control (CDC) has specific criteria for cleaning the rooms of patients with these illnesses. For example, the CDC requires that all hospital personnel wear a protective mask when they enter the rooms of patients having respiratory illnesses. There are other guidelines for patients with infected wounds and other infections in their bodies, as well as special procedures for patients with highly contagious diseases. These guidelines offer the greatest protection to both the environmental services worker and the patient.

The CDC's 1987 recommendation for universal blood and body fluid precautions states that all patients are to be considered potentially infective. Thus all health care workers are required to wear gloves when dealing with patient blood and body fluids or surfaces that could be contaminated by them.

Figure 3-5. Procedure for Cleaning Patient Room—Occupied (Approximate Time: 10 Minutes)

Procedure:	#4
Effective:	1/67
Revisions:	10/84
	1/85
	4/86
	9/87
	5/88
	5/89
Responsibility:	Environmental Assistants I and II.
Purpose:	To provide a safe, clean, and attractive environment conducive to a speedy recovery; to prevent cross-infection from the inanimate environment
Equipment:	1 clean damp cloth wrung out in germicidal solution, plastic bags, wet mop, 1 clean dry cloth, disposable gloves, doodle duster, mop bucket, prescribed germicidal solution
Special Requirements:	Germicidal solution must be changed in mop bucket after 3–4 patient rooms have been cleaned.

Procedure	Key Points
1. Damp dust and dry all the following: Top of overbed table Top of front of bedside cabinet Telephone and cords TV control and call button Column and base of overbed table Lamp and cord Switch plates—connection plates Windowsill Air conditioner Chairs and hassock Flower table Thermostats Door handle and hinges	a. Put on gloves. b. Clean first four elements in order. The other elements may be done in any order. While wiping refold cloth to use clean side. Place soiled cleaning cloths in plastic bag on cart.
2. Empty and reline wastebaskets.	Place not more than three extra bags in the basket before relining.
3. Dust mop floor, moving furniture where necessary.	
4. Wet mop floor and half of corridor outside of room, as you come out of the door. Continue to next room door on the same side of corridor.	Wet mop should be wrung as dry as possible to prevent slipping.

Note: Be sure to place wet-floor signs in doorway of patient room.

The CDC further recommends that the best defense is being sure that environmental surfaces are not the source of a nosocomial (hospital-acquired) infection. The best way to ensure this is to make certain that all surfaces are washed and that plenty of "elbow grease" is used. Because most germs need food and moisture to survive, it is important that all foreign matter be removed from surfaces to make the environment as germfree as possible.

There are times when the nature of an illness, the condition of a patient, or the attitude of the staff is such that cleaning procedures beyond what would be considered reasonable are requested. At these times, the environmental services director must collaborate with his or her staff to determine what is feasible so as to meet the staff's concerns. It would also be extremely important to involve the infection control officer at this time so that an acceptable solution can be reached.

Figure 3-6. Environmental Assistant I Training Progress Checklist

St. Luke's Hospital
Milwaukee, Wisconsin

ENVIRONMENTAL ASSISTANT I TRAINING PROGRESS CHECKLIST
X-1966   Rev. 6/86

This checklist will help you and the Department keep track of your training as an Environmental Assistant. Our goal is to help you become certified by performing each of the elements listed on your own and on several separate occasions. You will be trained to perform each element according to procedure and to the acceptable level of quality as outlined in the department's written standards. upon reaching this goal and successfully completing the six week followup, you will receive a certificate of achievement.

EMPLOYEE'S NAME _____   DATE OF HIRE _____

DAY 1: INITAL AND DATE AS MATERIAL IS PRESENTED AND DISCUSSED		
☐ BODY MECHANICS (VIDEO)	☐ EMERGENCY PREPAREDNESS PLAN	☐ JOB DESCRIPTION	☐ CALLING IN/EMPLOYEE ABSENCE POLICIES
☐ GUEST RELATIONS	☐ DAY 1 ☐ DAY 10 FIRE EXTINGUISHER (VIDEO)	☐ DAY 1 ☐ DAY 10	☐ INFECTION CONTROL (VIDEO)
☐ DRESS/UNIFORM & APPEARANCE POLICY	☐ INSPECT. SHT. WRITTEN STDS.	☐ THINGS TO KNOW	☐ TOUR
☐ CODE 4 ☐ SAFETY MEASURES		

ELEMENT	CART SET UP AND CLEANING (DAY 2-5)	MOPPING (DAY 2-5)	PT. ROOM (DAY: 2-1ST 4-2ND)	EXAM RM. (DAY: 4-1ST 2-2ND)	BATH-ROOMS (DAY 2)	UTILITY ROOMS (DAY 2)	OFFICES (DAY 2)	DIS-MISSAL UNIT (DAY 3)	FREQUENCY SCHEDULE (DAY 3-5)	SERVICE CLOSET (DAY 3)	ISOLATION CLEANING (DAY 4)	TRASH AND LINEN (DAY 5)	WALL WASHING (DAY 5)	WINDOW WASHING (DAY 5)
READS & DISCUSSES WRITTEN PROCEDURE (DATE)														
AREA PROCEDURE DEMONSTRATED														
EMPLOYEE'S HANDS ON PRACTICE														
EMPLOYEE OBSERVED INDICATING STEPS IN PROCEDURE BY NO. (USE COMMENT SECTION)														
REVIEW OF WRITTEN STANDARDS														
EMPLOYEE DEMONSTRATES COMPETENCE (DATES) — 1ST SHIFT	4x	3x	5x	2x	5x	2x	2x	3x	5x	3x	1x	1x	3x	3x
EMPLOYEE DEMONSTRATES COMPETENCE (DATES) — 2ND SHIFT	4x	1x	2x	5x	5x	1x	5x	3x	5x	3x	1x	1x	1x	1x
WEEK 2 FOLLOW-UP	1x	1x	2x	2x	3x	1x	2x	2x	3x	1x	ORAL REV. 1x	1x	1x	1x
WEEK 4 FOLLOW-UP	1x	1x	2x	2x	2x	1x	2x	1x	2x	1x	ORAL REV. 1x	1x	1x	1x
WEEK 6 FOLLOW-UP	1x	1x	1x	1x	1x	1x	1x	1x	1x	1x	ORAL REV. 1x	1x	1x	1x

SEE REVERSE SIDE

Source: Reprinted, with permission, from Saint Luke's Medical Center, Milwaukee.

Quality Assurance

An active quality assurance system for environmental services can provide feedback to employees, supply the manager with a measurable performance of the department, and ensure that patients and visitors are getting the best service possible. Cleanliness standards should be established for the department (figure 3-7).

Although routine, informal inspections are an important step in quality assurance, it is essential that formal, written inspections be done on a regular basis. An inspection form (figure 3-8) is used to record all items that are to be inspected and their condition at the time of inspection.

Evaluations of how well the employee completed the assigned tasks will enable the inspector, the department head, and the employee to become part of the evaluation process. These evaluations provide an excellent, nonsubjective component of the employee's work record and can be used in performance reviews.

Recognition is a vital part of any department leader's responsibility, and it is extremely important in the environmental services department. Positive feedback and recognition lets staff members know that they are appreciated. These efforts will increase employee morale and confidence, which will be evident to incoming guests and patients.

Figure 3-7. Housekeeping Standards for Quality Control

I. Floors

A. Tile

1. The floor is clean and free of dust, marks, and spots.
2. The floor has a visible, overall shine that is rich and easily recognizable.
3. There is no wax or dirt buildup anywhere on the floor.
4. There are no excessive spots, scuffs, or scratches on traffic lanes, around furniture, and at pivot points.
5. Corners are clean and free of soil or dust.
6. There are no spots, scratches, or scuffs in nontraffic areas.
7. There are no heavy black markings.
8. The floor is free of litter.
9. The floor does not need mopping.
10. The floor does not need stripping or scrubbing.
11. The floor finish is framed neatly around the room or down the center of the corridor.
12. The threshold is free of dirt, buildup, and overlap marks.

B. Baseboards

1. The baseboard, corners, and top edge are clean and free of dust, wax buildup, and soil film.
2. There are no signs of improper mopping, scrubbing, or vacuum-shampooing techniques.

C. Carpet

1. The carpet is clean and free of dust, lint, litter, and spots.
2. The carpet pile is even and shows no marks, crushing, or footprints.
3. Edges, corners, and around furniture legs are free of dust, lint, and spots.
4. The carpet does not need vacuuming.
5. The carpet has no spots or stains.
6. The carpet appears to be in a well-maintained condition.

II. Walls

A. Wall Surface

1. The walls are clean and free of spots, dust, streaks, and smudges.
2. There are no marks on the wall due to furniture or equipment.
3. There are no fingerprints around light switches or on door frames.

Figure 3-8. Housekeeping Inspection Quality Control Form

St. Luke's Medical Center
Milwaukee, WI 53215

HOUSEKEEPING INSPECTION
QUALITY CONTROL
X-1087 Rev. 2/88

AREA # *013*		AREA INSPECTED *HCD*	DATE *2/25/91*

☐ KITCHEN	☐ CORRIDOR	☐ OFFICE	☐ ELEVATOR	☒ PT. BATH	☐ DISMISSAL UNIT	☐ VENDING ROOM
	☐ LOBBY	☐ STAIRWAY	☐ PT. ROOM	☐ PUBLIC BATH	☐ EXAM ROOMS	☐ LOCKER ROOM

PERCENTAGE STANDARD OF CLEANLINESS **90** %   EMPLOYEE *Jane D.*   INSPECTED BY *Bob*

	ELEMENTS	S	U	ELEMENTS	S	U
FLOORS	TILE / CARPET			BASEBOARDS / CORNERS	✓	
	SHOWER	✓		THRESHOLDS	✓	
WALLS	WALL	✓		HINGES / DOOR FRAME	✓	
	VENTS	✓		DIVIDERS		
	STAINLESS STEEL					
WINDOWS	GLASS			WINDOW COVERINGS		
	FRAME / SILLS / LEDGES			HARDWARE		
	AIR CONDITIONING VENTS					
CEILINGS	LIGHT FIXTURES			VENTS	✓	
	CEILINGS					
FURNISHINGS	WASTE CONTAINERS / STEP ON CANS		✓	BEDSIDE CABINET		
	TABLES			OVERBED TABLE		
	DESKS			SHOWER CURTAIN	✓	
	CHAIRS			CUBICLE CURTAINS / TRACKS		
	TELEVISION			LAMPS / SHADES / CORDS		
	TV CONTROL / CALL BUTTON	✓		LOCKERS		
	TELEPHONE AND CORD			FILE CABINETS		
	BED / FRAMES / SPRINGS			SUCTION GAUGES		
	MONITOR			REFRIGERATOR		
	LINEN CARTS					
	CAMERAS					
	MICROWAVE / STOVE					
FIXTURES	MIRROR & FRAME / MED. CABINET	✓		WATER FOUNTAINS		
	MIRROR LIGHT / OVERBED LIGHT	✓		THERMOSTAT		
	SINK	✓		PICTURES / MIRRORS		
	TOILET	✓		ROOM SIGNS		
	URINALS			RAILINGS		
	TUB / SHOWER	✓		FIRE EXTINGUISHER / ALARMS		
	SOAP / TOWEL / SANITARY DISP.	✓		STANDPIPES		
	SHELVES / HOLDERS / BARS	✓		CLOCKS		
	SPRAYER / HOSE		✓	STAINLESS STEEL		
	FAUCETS / PIPES / SHOWER HEAD	✓		CLOSET FLOOR		
	CONNECTION & SWITCH PLATES	✓				
	CLOSET SHELF					
	COMMENTS					

Employee Signature _*Jane*_

Source: Reprinted, with permission, from Saint Luke's Medical Center, Milwaukee.

☐ Summary

Today's environmental services department must have a well-trained, ambitious staff. Its leadership must be skilled in human and interpersonal relations. The ability to locate, interpret, and follow specific guidelines, codes, and laws is also essential.

The value of a well-functioning environmental services department can be measured in the good guest relations that come from a well-maintained building, the high morale and excellent performance of the staff, the efficiency of its operation, and, finally, the comfort and goodwill of the people the facility serves—the patients.

☐ References and Bibliography

Joint Commission on Accreditation of Healthcare Organizations. *Accreditation Manual for Hospitals.* Oakbrook Terrace, IL: JCAHO, 1990.

Hazard Communication Standard: OSHA Final Rule (29 CFR 1910.1200). Published in *Federal Register,* 51:31877, 1986.

The MHA Recycling & Conservation Guide. Minneapolis: Minnesota Hospital Association, 1990.

Morbidity and Mortality Weekly Report Supplement 36(25), Aug. 31, 1987.

Resource Conservation and Recovery Act of 1976. Public Law 94-580. October 21, 1976.

State of Wisconsin, 1989 Wisconsin Act 335. Enacted: April 27, 1990. Published: May 10, 1990.

Chapter 4
Security

Sherman G. McGill, Jr.

☐ Overview

Health care administrators are often unaware of the devastating impact that inadequate or negligent security practices could have on their facilities. This chapter offers information and insight on how facilities can take positive and substantive action to ensure that they have a viable security and loss prevention program.

In response to the escalating number of lawsuits and subsequent court judgments alleging negligent or inadequate security, facilities should closely monitor and evaluate their security and loss prevention programs. Even though a facility may not be experiencing a high number of incidents, management should always be aware that an adverse incident can occur at any time. Facilities must have a security plan predicated on the reasonable expectation that such a situation may happen. Failure to do so may form the basis for a lawsuit charging inadequate or negligent security practice.

A case in point involved the tragic death of Dr. Kathryn Hinnant, a 33-year-old pathologist at Bellevue Hospital in New York City. On January 7, 1989, Dr. Hinnant was raped and murdered in her office by a homeless vagrant. According to an article that appeared in *Hospital Security and Safety Management* (May 1989), Bellevue Hospital was "caught in an avalanche of negative publicity." Dr. Hinnant's husband filed a $25 million lawsuit against the hospital and New York City for inadequate security.

Security is also needed for other reasons besides protection of employees. It is estimated that loss of supplies because of theft, pilferage, and waste may account for as much as 20 percent of all health care costs. This loss is a substantial item in the cost of operating any medical care facility regardless of size or location. To reduce the loss of assets, health care facilities need to develop effective countermeasures (Rusting, 1987).

A comprehensive security program should be designed to provide for the protection of patients, staff, and visitors. Proactive programs to reduce liability and protect the loss of hospital assets translate into sound business practice.

Parts of this chapter were reprinted, with permission, from *Hospital Security and Safety Management* and from books published by Rusting Publications.

☐ Department Head Responsibilities

Implementation of a security program is the responsibility of the department head. This individual should work closely with administration to clearly define the authority and responsibilities of the department. When designing a comprehensive security structure for the facility, four major categories should be included:

- Prevention
- Detection
- Response
- Security education and training

Prevention plans include individual or integrated plans that deal with areas such as lock and key control, infant kidnapping, security of funds, and narcotics. A variety of protective measures can be planned to provide protection against the various forms of thefts and other threats facing the facility.

Detection plans should be addressed by such items as locking schedules and patrol plans. Other means of detection, such as inventories, audits, and inspections, may be included in separate prevention plans as well. The use of closed-circuit television (CCTV) and intrusion detection should be addressed in this plan.

Response should be included for routine matters in the other plans. Some specialized response plans are required, but they should be limited to dangerous incidents. For example, a specialized response plan may focus on bomb threats, fire evacuation, a hostage crisis, and so forth.

Security education and training cannot be overly stressed as a means of asset protection and reduction of liability. The training program should specifically include knowledge of local law and management of violent behavior. The training of security personnel could become a major focal point should civil litigation be filed. If a loss or injury is caused by security personnel who are inadequately trained, management may incur legal exposure through vicarious liability in an area known as training negligence (Turner, 1988, pp. 26, 56).

☐ Department Head Qualifications

Many hospitals are combining safety, security, and risk management functions. The individual selected to be the security director should have excellent written and oral communication skills. A competent security director will need these attributes to successfully lobby for and implement asset protection programs that many employees and staff members may find unpalatable.

The security director should also be capable of working in conjunction with the human resources department to ensure that proper preemployment screening methods are utilized. These efforts may help to ward off charges of negligent hiring, retention, and training.

The American Society of Industrial Security (ASIS) and the International Association for Healthcare Security and Safety (IAHSS) have developed professional standards and testing programs that attest to an individual's mastery of the profession. The Certified Protection Professional Program is administered by the ASIS and the Certified Healthcare Protection Administrator by the IAHSS.

The director of security should also be an effective planner. The security functions to be implemented should be clearly defined in a policy and procedures manual.

☐ Organization of the Department and Staffing

When a health care facility forms a security department, it is imperative that a comprehensive security and loss prevention assessment be performed before manpower allocation is determined. Specifically, a program should be designed to manage identified vulnerabilities instead of hiring a security staff and then deciding what activities they will perform.

Organization of the security function can vary depending on the size of the facility and its operational requirements and the responsibilities of the security staff. For example, in a small facility, maintenance personnel on duty may be required to don their security hats and respond to situations that would usually be handled by security officers in larger health care facilities. Small facilities mainly rely on their staff and assistance from law enforcement agencies to handle security-related matters. Large facilities often employ sophisticated security measures that include a staff of extensively trained personnel.

The organizational structure of security departments can be broken down into operational and support sections. The operations division of a large facility may be staffed by a security supervisor on each shift, with a complement of officers reporting to that person. The supervisors may in turn report to a senior supervisor or the assistant director of security. The operations division would typically be responsible for conducting internal and external patrols, providing employee escorts, responding to calls for assistance, and taking security incident reports. Some facilities are large enough to have their own investigative section, and the individuals in this section may report either through the operations chain of command or directly to the director of security.

The support division may perform such functions as office administration, lock and key control, management of the identification badge program, lost and found, and so forth. In addition, the management of parking services may be associated with this section.

The security apparatus in smaller to medium-sized hospitals may comprise the director of security, possibly a senior supervisor, and a staff of four or five officers. In smaller departments, the staff usually perform both the operational and support functions.

Hospital administrators and security directors should be aware of potential staffing problems that presently confront the security industry and will continue to do so in the future. The largest single problem will be the shortage of qualified security officers. It is estimated that the number of people entering the labor market will grow by less than 1 percent per year in the 1990s (Naisbitt and Aburdene, 1990, p. 80). Compounding this problem for all occupations will be drug and alcohol abuse, criminal records, lack of education and training, and competition from other jobs. Hospital security organizations must view education and training as one of the strongest weapons available to them as they strive to keep pace with the challenges posed by a diminishing labor pool and changing technological advancements.

In-House versus Contract Security Services

When organizing or reorganizing a security department, management must determine whether to hire or retain an in-house security staff or utilize a contract security service. Providing high-quality security services is not so much a tactical decision as it is a business management objective.

There is little doubt that contract security services offer an advantage in terms of direct costs such as wages, payroll, taxes, benefits, training, equipment, and uniforms. However, other factors such as quality of service, level of training, loyalty, recruitment, and personnel screening programs must also be considered. Many companies that have made the decision to switch to contract services based solely on cost considerations have been disappointed when the level of service drops to compensate for the price. When considering whether to retain a contract security service, the questions in figure 4-1 will be helpful.

Some large facilities have opted to mix contract and in-house services. This method may offer cost savings and organizational flexibility in terms of redirecting the efforts of the director of security. This may free the director to devote more time to loss prevention initiatives rather than guard force management.

Figure 4-1. Questions for Deciding Whether to Use a Contract Security Service

---

1. What quantifiable cost benefits do I hope to achieve by using a guard service?
2. What specific objectives do I expect from a guard service?
3. What standards of performance do I expect from a guard service?
4. What steps need to be taken internally to increase the effectiveness of a guard service?

Management should also be aware that it cannot transfer all liability to the guard service. Management still may incur liability even though the security officer works for an independent contractor. The facility still may be exposed to liability based on:

- Negligence in hiring a guard company
- Control of the security officer
- Intentional torts committed by the security officer
- Delegation of inherently dangerous work

The following steps can be taken to reduce liability for the acts of a guard company:

- Conduct a careful, complete inquiry before hiring security guards or selecting a security guard company.
- Be sure the guard company has properly instructed its guards about detaining people and using force with respect to security incidents (use public law enforcement authorities) and has narrowly defined the guards' duties.
- Avoid entrusting the guards with inherently dangerous investigations. Use public law enforcement agencies in these situations.
- Add a clause to the written contract with guard service companies that indemnifies the facility against any liability resulting from the negligence of the guard company. This has value only to the extent that the guard company is financially sound (Rea, 1989).

Before deciding whether to use an outside contractor or develop an in-house department, facilities need to evaluate their available resources and select the service that best suits their needs.

☐ Specific Tasks Done within the Department

The mission of security departments should be to protect and serve the facility and its patients, visitors, and employees by performing the following functions:

- Protecting patients, visitors, and employees from harm and reasonable fear of harm
- Maintaining order, control, and safety in the facility's building(s) and on the campus
- Protecting personal and health care facility assets from theft, misuse, and vandalism
- Enforcing facility rules and regulations
- Conveying a professional image through actions conducive to good facility and community relations

To accomplish these goals, security officers perform the following tasks:

- Patrol all areas of the facility campus, including parking areas, on a regular basis. This may be done on foot, in a vehicle, or a combination of both.

- Provide access control through the lock and key program or electronic means such as card reader systems. Security in larger facilities is responsible for CCTV and alarm system monitoring. Security investigates intrusion into unauthorized areas.
- Assist in the enforcement of visiting regulations after hours.
- Initiate and implement package and parcel inspection as well as locker inspection programs. In addition, security staffs may be responsible for administering the patient valuables program.
- Investigate and document all thefts and suspected thefts, suspicious persons or activities, assaults, drug abuse, or any other action or matter that is deemed a threat to the well-being of patients, employees, or visitors.
- Provide escort services to employees and visitors upon request. Many larger facilities run shuttle services between the facility and parking areas.
- Participate in fire and disaster control operations.

□ Why Security Is Needed

There are many reasons why health care facilities need adequate security. After examining the issues of theft, pilferage, and waste, this section discusses damage awards, the increase in crime, and issues concerning the assurance of patient safety, including the legal precedents for providing security precautions and the consequences of inadequate security.

Theft, Pilferage, and Waste

Although a percentage of theft is perpetrated by patients and outsiders, most security analysts agree that the vast majority of theft is committed by facility employees. Approximately 3,000 items that are purchased by facilities can be used in the home (Colling, 1982, p. 41).

In fact, according to *Hospital Security*, it is estimated that as much as 20 percent of all hospital costs are attributed to losses from theft, pilferage, and waste. Other experienced security directors estimate the loss at $3,000 per bed per year (Colling, 1982).

Results from the Hollinger-Clark study, a comprehensive study of employee theft in the health care industry that appeared in *Theft in Hospitals and Nursing Homes* (Rusting, 1987, pp. 7-8, 17-19), underline the problems faced by the industry. The study was conducted by Richard Hollinger, Ph.D., funded by the U.S. Department of Justice, and supervised by the University of Minnesota.

Hollinger and his collaborator, John P. Clark, Ph.D., of the University of Minnesota, obtained their data from detailed questionnaires filled out by employees at all levels of health care facilities and retail and manufacturing facilities in the Minneapolis–St. Paul, Cleveland, and Dallas–Fort Worth areas. Over 2,000 employees at 21 health care facilities in these areas were surveyed.

The study revealed that one out of every three employees participating in the study admitted to stealing property (such as supplies or equipment), and 69 percent were guilty of stealing time (for example, using sick leave when not sick, arriving late, and leaving early).

Following are some other examples in the study.

- Twenty-seven percent said they took supplies (bandages, linens, and so forth) at least once a year, whereas 9 percent said they did so 4 to 12 times a year.
- Eight percent admitted to taking medicine intended for patients.
- Five percent confessed to stealing tools or equipment.
- Thirty-three percent admitted to taking sick leave when they were not sick.
- Three percent admitted to working under the influence of alcohol or drugs.

Theft of time is the second side of the loss coin for health care facilities, and it can add up to a considerable amount. According to an annual study done by Robert Half International, an executive recruitment firm, the average employee intentionally steals over four hours' worth of time a week in a typical year. This amounts to more than 10 percent of his or her salary and benefits. When the number of persons employed in the health care field is considered, time theft rivals property theft as a serious loss problem. In effect, employers are hiring 10 percent more employees than needed to compensate for the lost time.

An example of how property theft and lost time affect facilities can be found in *Theft in Hospitals and Nursing Homes* (Rusting, 1987). Rusting estimates that in a 300-bed facility with approximately $52 million a year in net service revenues and $51 million in operating expenses, $17 million could be spent on supplies and related expenses (33 percent of operating expenses). Using a 20 percent loss estimate, the facility could be spending more than $3.4 million as a result of employee theft, which amounts to more than three times its operating surplus. Alternatively, if the more conservative rate of $3,000 per bed is used to estimate loss, the amount of property stolen over any given year can be as high as $900,000.

The same health care facility also spends $27 million in salaries, wages, and benefits for its 1,300 employees (53 percent of operating expenses). The average amount spent per employee is $21,000 a year. If time theft (according to the Robert Half International Study) equals 10 percent, losses to the facility would amount to $2.7 million a year.

There are many ways to prevent or control theft, pilferage, and waste. These are discussed in the program evaluation section near the end of this chapter.

Damage Awards and the Increase in Crime

A viable security and loss prevention program will play a critical role in protecting health care institutions against financial losses resulting from damage awards. Juries often award judgments based on the standards of reasonableness of the security program and the doctrine of foreseeability of adverse incidents.

Courts have also maintained that there is a *duty*, or implied contract, between the hospital and the patient that ensures the patient's safety. In negligence law, *duty* is the basis of liability. The law allows recovery from persons other than the perpetrator of the act. As a landlord, the health care facility may be held liable for the damages that result from criminal acts conducted on its property.

It is imperative that hospitals become more security conscious for several reasons. The National Crime Prevention Institute has stated that the number of civil cases alleging inadequate security has greatly increased the frequency and size of damage awards since the 1970s. Estimates for damages awarded in security negligence suits average $850,000 per case (Bottom, 1985, pp. 3–5).

According to a 1989 *Lipman Report* (p. 1) published by Guardsmark, Inc., the overall crime rate in the United States has risen for the fourth consecutive year. FBI-Uniform Crime Reports for 1988 indicate that violent crime such as murder, forcible rape, aggravated assault, and robbery increased 5 percent as a group.

Other data document an increase in crime. A 1989 survey of crime in health care facilities was conducted by the IAHSS. A total of 315 facilities from all 50 states responded to the survey. Table 4-1 shows the results of that survey.

Legal Precedents for Providing Security Precautions

In October 1988, the Nebraska Supreme Court reversed a trial court's decision dismissing a suit by a surgery patient against Lutheran General Hospital in Omaha. The patient stated that she was assaulted by a male employee of the facility. The suit charged that this action violated an implied contract whereby the facility agreed to provide a "private,

Table 4-1. Incident Totals and Percentages of Hospitals with Incidents, by Hospital Setting, 1989

	Unknown	Urban	Rural	Inner-City	Total
# of Hospitals % of Respondents	28 8.9	150 47.6	38 12.1	99 31.4	315 100.0
# of Arsons % of Hospitals	6 17.9	13 8.0	4 5.3	23 12.1	46 9.8
# of Sexual Assaults % of Hospitals	5 10.7	18 8.7	8 10.5	15 11.1	46 9.8
# of Assaults % of Hospitals	220 57.1	830 65.3	124 55.3	615 58.6	1789 61.3
# of Armed Robberies % of Hospitals	4 14.3	16 8.0	1 2.6	15 10.1	36 8.6
# of Kidnappings % of Hospitals	0 0.0	8[a] 2.7	3 5.3	4 4.0	15[a] 3.2
# of Homicides % of Hospitals	0 0.0	1 .7	0 0.0	0 0.0	1 0.0
# of Suicides % of Hospitals	5 17.9	12 6.0	3 5.3	5 4.0	25 6.3
# of Bomb Threats % of Hospitals	23 42.9	162 38.7	19 36.8	111 40.4	315 39.4
# of Thefts % of Hospitals	2,224 85.7	9,586 90.0	1,051[b] 81.6	9,703 97.0	22,564[b] 90.8
# of Lawsuits % of Hospitals	3 7.1	27[c] 7.3	4 7.9	15 11.1	49[c] 8.6
Mean FTE Change	+1.3	+2.4	+0.9	+1.8	+1.9

Source: International Association for Healthcare Security and Safety, 1989.

Note: The percentages of hospitals are not related to the actual numbers of occurrences listed directly above them. The percentages were obtained as the percentage of hospitals within each particular setting that reported at least one occurrence, whereas the actual numbers are the total counts of occurrences.

[a]One additional hospital reported 20 kidnappings.
[b]One additional hospital reported 10,000 thefts.
[c]One additional hospital reported 100 security-related lawsuits.

safe, secure environment for her care." The trial court upheld the hospital's contention that it followed proper procedure in hiring the employee and that at the time of the alleged incident, he was not performing his assigned duties. The Supreme Court found that "a patient is generally admitted to a hospital . . . under an implied obligation that he shall receive such reasonable care and attention for his safety as his mental and physical condition . . . may require." The court ordered the case to proceed to trial (*Hospital Security and Safety Management Newsletter*, June 1989).

The doctrine of foreseeability or absence of a prior, similar crime has often been used to defend against the lawsuits of victims of assaults, robberies, and so forth. Crime can no longer be regarded as a random or unforeseeable incident. Health care facilities should understand that inadequate security practices may increase the possibility of crimes being committed on their campuses.

Merryn Issacs et al. v. Huntington Memorial Hospital (1984) is a landmark decision relative to the doctrine of foreseeability. In that case, the California Supreme Court affirmed that a hospital may be held liable for inadequate security, in a ruling resulting from a parking lot assault of a physician in 1978. It further ruled that foreseeability may be established without proof of prior, similar incidents (Territo and Bromby, 1987, p. 80). The court noted that "a landowner should not get one free assault before he can be held liable for criminal acts which occur on his property." The ruling essentially states that health care facilities and other landowners may be held liable for criminal acts that occur on their property without evidence of prior, similar crimes on the property.

In another case, *Small v. McKennan Hospital* in Sioux Falls, South Dakota, a hospital employee was abducted from the hospital parking ramp in 1987 and was subsequently raped and murdered. Although the hospital maintained that no similar incidents had occurred, evidence was presented that proved there was criminal activity on or around the ramp. The trial court judge ruled in favor of the hospital, using the narrow interpretation of the "prior, similar" rule. However, the State Supreme Court followed the California ruling and returned the case to the jury.

Lawsuits brought regarding security practices may also result in punitive damage awards, where the actions complained of are of a sufficiently egregious nature. In many parts of the country, punitive damage awards are not covered by insurance and, therefore, must be paid by the health care facility. Awards may be avoided if the facility can demonstrate that it had security measures in place at the time an incident occurred. However, many times it is difficult and costly for a facility to prove that it was providing sufficient security precautions. The three security measures most often cited by courts when determining a business's liability are inadequate exterior lighting, not having fencing that surrounds the perimeter of the property, and a lack of private security guards.

The Florida District Court of Appeals stated in the case of *Ten Associates v. Brunsen* (1986) that even if security practices are proven to be inadequate and warrant compensatory damages, they may suffice to ward off a claim for punitive damages. In the *Brunsen* case, the appellate court overturned a verdict for punitive damages because the defendant landlord made an effort, albeit a negligent one, to control on-premises crime. Predicated on this significant but little-known Florida appellate decision, a business demonstrating a concern for safety and public well-being may be able to insulate itself from potentially large punitive damage awards.

Consequences of Inadequate Security

Case law clearly indicates that health care facilities have a duty to provide prudent and reasonable security precautions. Failure to act upon or satisfy this duty may lead to punitive or exemplary damage awards. Even though security operations may be perceived as costly, they are essential in this litigious environment. Awards of damages can cause serious and, in some cases, fatal economic blows to even thriving businesses (Anthony and Thornburg, 1989).

Adverse security-related incidents are often viewed in an emotional light. As such, the perception that a health care facility is negligent or has inadequate security can be extremely costly. Not only may the courts award a multimillion-dollar judgment, but the institution's reputation in the community may be severely tarnished as well. This is doubly compounded because the facility's staff may become fearful and suffer morale problems.

Dissatisfaction with security at many health care facilities is becoming a major factor in their ability to recruit and keep nurses. Nurses are extremely concerned about security, especially in large urban facilities (*Hospital Security and Safety Management Newsletter*, Mar. 1989).

Negative publicity related to poor security can have a major impact on the bottom line. If prospective patients fear for their safety, they will choose a facility that can provide the level of security they seek.

The Bellevue murder case, infant kidnappings, and the other cases cited herein are excellent examples of the profound impact that security programs may have on health care facilities. Not only does a bad security record diminish employee morale, it has far-reaching consequences within the community as well.

☐ Ensuring Adequate Security

The key to avoiding liability for security practices is to take steps to provide for reasonable and adequate security and to make sure the measures are well documented. Oftentimes if a procedure is not documented, it is not considered by the courts to have been done. Not all health care facilities need or require full-time security staffs, but they must have security policies and procedures in place.

Health care facilities throughout the country are coping with severe budgetary restrictions, and some facilities may be tempted to cut their security departments simply because they are viewed as not producing revenue. However, this strategy can backfire if patients do not regard the facility as safe. A better strategy is to use the existence of a professional security staff as both a marketing and recruitment tool.

☐ Equipment and Technology

Labor dollars account for a large percentage of operational costs in security departments. Many health care security departments have realized that it is practical and cost-effective to use technology and procedural methods to reduce labor costs. For example, through the use of CCTV or electronic access control, one security officer can supervise activity at numerous locations.

Machines can monitor many areas simultaneously, operate in hostile environments, work invisibly, and cover wide areas. Alarms become the eyes and ears of security officers, and CCTV and a video recorder can provide a record of what transpired. It remains the job of professional security officers to evaluate and respond based on what the machines have reported.

Security components that are often utilized in health care facilities include:

- CCTV cameras
- Electronic access control devices, such as card readers or digital keypads
- Door alarm/door status monitoring systems
- Fire alarm panels
- Intrusion detection sensors

These devices can be configured to stand alone or as a fully integrated and distributed network capable of monitoring all systems at the same time.

Security technology changes at a very rapid pace, and this trend shows no sign of ceasing. Many systems are now computer based; therefore, the operator must be computer literate. It is important that security directors stay abreast of the type of equipment on the market and its capabilities.

Security hardware is not cheap, and the selection of inferior or outdated equipment can have tremendous operational and financial consequences for the department and the health care facility. For example, if a facility plans to integrate several types of electronic systems, it must be determined at the outset whether the systems will interface with one another. The purchase of systems that will not "talk to one another" as planned is a very costly mistake.

The integration of technology into protection plans is a sound business decision. However, management must be very careful in their selection process to ensure that the hardware they purchase will perform as advertised and in the manner that the end user specifies.

☐ Safety and Compliance

Health care facilities must be concerned with the safety of employees, visitors, and patients. They should not only be concerned about accident prevention, but other aspects of safety as well. For example, a comprehensive risk assessment program should include the following security elements:

- Security programs should include assessments of the ways staff, patients, and visitors are being provided protection; a survey that accounts for materials, equipment, and physical assets; management of the risks inherent in the facility; and an assessment of the security of information and information systems within the organization.
- The security program should be consistent with the needs of the organization. It should consider such variables as location and environment, vehicular and pedestrian traffic, local police response and capabilities, and the security needs of patients, employees, visitors, and vendors.
- A manager should be appointed to oversee the elements of the security program.
- An appropriate method for identifying employees should be established. The facility should consider using identification badges for this purpose.
- Key and lock systems should be standardized to provide consistent security for information and equipment. The key system should be designed to provide optimum retrieval and tracking of issued keys, as well as for anticipated expansion. This system should be evaluated regularly and updated as necessary.
- The physical security of medical records as well as electronic password security should be provided to protect medical information systems and similar electronic information systems.

Joint Commission standards place a great deal of emphasis on evaluating the impact of patient care and safety. As a result, a security program that addresses concerns regarding patients, visitors, personnel, and property should be an integral component of the overall risk management strategy.

Health care administrators wanting additional information on health care security standards can contact the IAHSS (see appendix C). This organization has also developed the Hospital Security Officer Basic Training Certification Standard and the Supervisory Development Standard. Both these actions are the first of their kind within the industry.

Health care administrators must be cognizant of what law courts are saying about inadequate or negligent security practices. The specter of increased liability for failure to initiate protective safeguards, coupled with staggering losses, certainly makes security programs essential and cost-justifiable.

☐ Program Evaluation

Administrators can evaluate and make informed decisions about their programs by commissioning a comprehensive security/loss prevention assessment for their facilities. This evaluation may be completed by the director of security if qualified, or by an independent security/loss prevention consultant.

A security/loss prevention assessment has several objectives:

- To delineate an adequate security program that provides for the protection and safety of patients, visitors, employees, and staff
- To deter and reduce the incidence of theft, pilferage, and waste of company assets
- To ascertain the true extent of such activity
- To address potential litigation resulting from allegations of inadequate or negligent security

The success of the program can be measured through a survey that should provide an appraisal of:

- The threats or risks affecting the assets to be safeguarded
- The likelihood or probability of those threats becoming actual loss events
- The impact on the facility if the threat is realized

The survey should provide a comprehensive evaluation of the facility, its hours of operation, the local crime rate (crime profile), and other environmental conditions that will affect the foreseeability factor that juries take into account when a crime is committed.

The physical and procedural security measures (if any) at the facility should be evaluated and recommendations made for additions or modifications to increase efficiency and cost-effectiveness. The surveyor should assist the facility administrator in developing and documenting a plan for "adequate and reasonable" security.

A record of the security assessment and the protective measures taken should be maintained. These records constitute a protection portfolio. Although they may not bar litigation entirely, they will be valuable evidence in the event of a negligent security lawsuit.

In addition to the previously mentioned items, the survey should provide specific recommendations such as those included in figure 4-2. These are but a few of the recommendations that can be made to improve a facility's security program.

The survey should be the foundation upon which intelligent, cost-justifiable, and informed business decisions are made. The survey will provide administrators or responsible managers with an in-depth analysis of current strong points and shortcomings and a method by which to facilitate proactive and positive change.

Addressing the Problems of Theft, Pilferage, and Waste

The control of theft, pilferage, and waste represents one of the best opportunities for health care administrators to reduce their operating expenses. Many issues that evolve into security matters are actually management problems. Management must realize that security is everyone's responsibility. Security directors and their staffs should become an integral part of the overall facility loss prevention/risk management program.

Health care facilities should formulate a specific antitheft policy and make sure that all department heads are responsible and accountable for implementing programs that reduce theft and pilferage in their respective areas. An example cited in the Hollinger-Clark study showed that facilities with a strong antitheft policy, and those that practice preemployment screening, had a lower incidence of theft.

The security director should work with department managers to educate them about employee theft and loss prevention techniques. The problem should be addressed in a proactive manner rather than simply in reaction to a crime problem. In addition, it should be understood that many documented cases of white-collar crime such as fraud, embezzlement, and kickbacks occur at health care facilities. These crimes are typically committed by administrators, controllers, purchasing managers, business office managers, and so forth. Thus, security staff and department managers need to be alert for white-collar crime incidents as well.

McGill

Figure 4-2. Security Assessment Overview: Example of Recommendations

1. Security operations management
   A. Proprietary vs. contract
   B. Prevention plans
   C. Detection plans
   D. Response plans
   E. Security education and training
   F. Departmental automation

2. Perimeter security
   A. Clearly defined property boundary
   B. Fencing
   C. Low shrubbery

3. Keys: issue and control
   A. Documented policy
   B. Employee accountability
   C. Security of keys
   D. Tracking
   E. Retrieval

4. Information security
   A. Medical records
   B. Computer security

5. Personnel security
   A. Preemployment screening and background investigation
   B. Security awareness and education
   C. Driver risk control program
   D. Preemployment and postemployment drug testing policy

6. Parking area security, signage, and protective lighting
   A. Control point
   B. Patrol
   C. Surveillance
   D. Proper illumination levels (footcandles)
   E. Signage/discharge

7. Access control and building security
   A. Lockdown schedules
   B. Electronic access control
   C. Employee badge/identification system
   D. Visitor/vendor control
   E. Key and lock systems

8. CCTV and alarm systems
   A. Proper placement
   B. Lens selection
   C. Installation
   D. High-vulnerability areas
   E. Deterrence factor

9. Theft and pilferage
   A. Antitheft policy
   B. Inventory controls
   C. Package inspection
   D. Locker inspection
   E. Patient valuables

Administrators should take a hard look at what efforts are being undertaken to control inventory and reduce theft. The answer does not always lie with throwing dollars at the problem. The response should be proportionate to the threat. In other words, a $100,000 expenditure for a security system (hardware) is not required if solid policies and procedures can be implemented that will rectify the problem.

☐ Summary

Budgetary constraints in the public sector, coupled with a nationwide increase in crime, have forced many traditional police functions to shift to private security forces. As they deal with their own financial crises, health care institutions are charged with providing for the safety and security of their patients, employees, and visitors. There should be no misunderstanding that the courts have imposed a duty on health care facilities to protect "invitees" on their campuses. The liability that these institutions face as a result of inadequate or negligent security, coupled with the negative impact of theft, pilferage, and waste, represents a potentially devastating threat.

These threats command dynamic response from management. Health care facilities should have a security/loss prevention program that is based on sound economic and security management principles. To avoid litigation and loss of valuable company assets, a reasonable and prudent program must be in place.

☐ References and Bibliography

Anthony, A. J., and Thornburg, F. F. Liability lessons: security on trial. *Security Management Magazine* (Arlington, VA) 33(2):41–46, Feb. 1989.

The Bellevue murder; could it happen in your hospital? *Hospital Security and Safety Management* 10(1):6, May 1989.

Bottom, N. R. *Security Loss Control Negligence.* Columbia, MD: Hanrow Press, 1985.

Colling, R. Y. *Hospital Security,* 2nd ed. Stoneham, MA: Butterworth Publishers, 1982.

Crime reaches unprecedented levels. *The Lipman Report.* Memphis, TN: Guardsmark, July 1989.

Legal trend update: why hospitals face growing risks. *Hospital Security and Safety Management* 9(9):7, Jan. 1989.

Naisbitt, J., and Aburdene, P. *Megatrends 2000.* New York City: William Morrow & Co., 1990.

Nurses spell out concerns about hospital security. *Hospital Security and Safety Management* 9(11):1, Mar. 1989.

Rea, K. V. Avoiding a catch-22, liability lessons. *Security Management Magazine* (Arlington, VA), 33(7):39–41, July 1989.

Rusting, R. *Theft in Hospitals and Nursing Homes.* Port Washington, NY: Rusting Publications, 1987.

Security. Des Plaines, IL: Cahners Publishing, June 1988, p. 17.

Somerson, I. S. Managing your guard dollars. *Security Management Magazine* (Arlington, VA) 32(1):91–95, Jan. 1988.

Ten Associates v. Brunsen, 492 So. 2d 1149 (1986).

Territo, L., and Bromby, M. L. *Hospital and College Security Liability.* Columbia, MD: Hanrow Press, 1987.

Turner, J. T. *Handbook of Hospital Security and Safety.* Rockville, MD: Aspen Publishers, 1988.

Two states differ on hospital's implied contract for patient security. *Hospital Security and Safety Management* 10(2):14, June 1989.

Walsh, T. J., and Healy, R. *Protection of Assets Manual.* Santa Monica, CA: The Merritt Company, 1988.

Chapter 5
Safety

Linda F. Chaff

☐ Overview

Safety has traditionally been associated with fire prevention or slippery floors, but the concept of safety within today's health care facility must encompass much more than that. Very few businesses provide service 24 hours a day, 365 days a year, with no downtime for holidays or untimely interruptions. Not only are health care facilities responsible for providing employees with a safe working environment, but they are entrusted with the safety of patients, visitors, and volunteers as well. By allowing hazardous conditions to exist or practicing unsafe acts, the health care facility is creating a potentially dangerous environment for each life it touches.

Today's health care industry is faced with challenging and complex issues that are forcing health care facilities to cope with a range of safety concerns unimagined only a few years ago. Among these new health care issues are the consequences that accompany the benefits brought by advancements in technology. Sophisticated machinery and tools such as lasers are introducing new risks to the industry at the same time they are enhancing treatment for patients.

AIDS is an excellent example of a pressing health care issue that was not faced by our country a decade ago. It is the facility's responsibility to provide high-quality care for patients with this illness and at the same time ensure the best possible safety conditions for employees.

Other diverse issues such as shifting demographics, an aging population requiring specialized care, and increasing competition also work together to affect the role safety plays within a health care facility. Unsafe conditions can result in bad publicity that can easily damage a facility's competitive position, whereas safe conditions can enhance patient care and attract new patients.

Health care facilities also face the challenge of meeting various safety standards required by the growing number of governmental and voluntary regulatory agencies. As facilities increasingly rely on hazardous chemicals, the need for additional monitoring programs increases. To keep pace with these changes and growth areas, it is important to keep abreast of the rapid changes in the standards required by these agencies, which are discussed in chapter 6.

Liability is a pressing concern for health care facilities. Patients were once reluctant to sue their neighborhood health care facility or doctor. Now, however, with the belief that medical attention is less personal, litigation has become a frequent option for those patients who feel their treatment was inadequate or negligent. This includes accidents, such as burns and falls, that are not directly related to medical care. However, well-adhered-to safety measures can prevent accidents that could otherwise result in monetary losses.

As health care facilities implement and embrace effective safety programs, the results will become evident in many areas. Employee accidents can be reduced, along with worker's compensation claims and lost work time. As facilities comply with regulations, citations and penalties from regulatory agencies, such as the Occupational Safety and Health Administration (OSHA), can also be avoided. A comprehensive safety program will also help maintain accreditation by the Joint Commission on Accreditation of Healthcare Organizations (Joint Commission). As staff members work together as a team to make the facility a safer place to work, stay, or visit, morale and productivity will increase and liability for accidents and injuries will decrease.

☐ Department Head Responsibilities

Making the health care facility safe is everyone's responsibility, but to ensure that a high-quality job is done, one individual must oversee and coordinate this process. That individual is either the facility's safety director, a budgeted appointment, or its safety officer, a volunteer position filled by a staff member.

Whether the facility has a full-time safety director or a staff member serving as the safety officer, that individual must understand the important role he or she plays within the facility's overall safety program. The Joint Commission specifically requires the administration to appoint a safety officer who is qualified either by training or experience.

One issue that often arises when the administration examines the safety director's role in the facility is need versus cost. However, in a survey conducted by the National Safety Council, 75 percent of the facilities responded that they do not conduct a safety program cost–benefit analysis (National Safety Council, 1990). Periodically, an administration may feel that it is difficult to measure the direct effects of a safety program, yet a close examination of the responsibilities of the safety officer or director will show otherwise. The administration's acceptance and understanding of the responsibilities of that position will enable the administration and the safety director to establish a positive working relationship.

The safety director's main objective is to prevent accidents. An accident that was prevented will never appear on a report or as a statistic. However, a qualified and experienced director should possess the skills not only to reduce risks in a number of areas (figure 5-1), but also to provide evidence of his or her work.

The safety director's overall role is that of leader of the safety management program—developing, implementing, and monitoring it. He or she works closely with the safety committee to review accident trends, conduct inspections, keep policies and procedures current and effective, maintain a liaison with departments, serve on multiple facility committees, coordinate fire and disaster drills, and help design motivational programs for safety. To achieve these goals, the safety director works closely with the administration to provide and receive input and suggestions that will enhance the safety program. The program's impact should demonstrate these efforts.

The safety director should serve as a resource for all safety concerns and should be guided by a current job description. After reviewing the safety director's scope of responsibilities, it is quickly evident that one person cannot be entirely responsible for the facility's safety program. The scope and formality of a hospital's safety program will depend on the size of the facility and the nature of the potential risks. Large, complex medical

Figure 5-1. Areas of Responsibility for Safety Directors

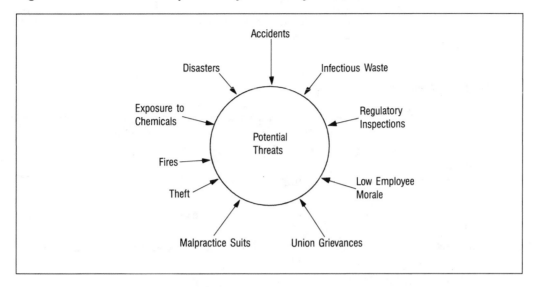

centers may have a department that includes both a safety director and safety officers; however, most facilities will be staffed only with a safety director.

The safety director relies on the cooperation and support of the other department heads, employees, and the safety committee to achieve a successful safety program. Most of the responsibility for safety is handled by each department head on a daily basis.

It is difficult for the safety director to identify an individual department's specific needs. As the various departments work together to promote a better image of safety within the health care facility, the safety director serves as a resource for each department, answering safety questions or establishing training programs. Once the department's needs have been identified, the safety director can help produce targeted safety programs designed to correct any predetermined problems, such as slips and falls, needle punctures, lock-out/tag-out procedures in maintenance, or chemotherapy waste procedures in pharmacy.

☐ Members of the Safety Committee

The safety committee should include members who are professionally qualified and are capable of developing, implementing, and maintaining a comprehensive, facilitywide safety program. The Joint Commission requires that the committee be composed of representatives from various departments and areas, including administration, clinical services, and support services.

A typical safety committee could include the following members:

- Administrative representative
- Medical staff representative
- At least one nursing representative
- Director of maintenance (or engineering, or both)
- Supervisory representative (one to three, on rotation)
- Director of housekeeping
- Director of dietary
- Human resources representative
- Safety officer
- Labor representative (if there is a union)
- Three nonsupervisory employees (rotated periodically)

☐ Specific Tasks Related to Safety

Understanding the following diverse aspects of safety will help the administration to have a better relationship with the safety director, the safety committee, and the various department heads.

Activities of the Safety Committee

One of the ways to make a serious commitment to ensuring a safe environment for patients, visitors, and employees is to understand and support the facility's safety committee. The basic goal of the committee is to serve the hospital and make it a safer place for everyone.

To achieve this goal the safety committee has four objectives:

1. Provide the program director and/or chief executive officer (CEO) with technical support
2. Review submitted materials and develop safety policies for presentation to the administration for action
3. Create and promote a facilitywide concern for safety
4. Serve as a safety resource and advisory group

A clear understanding of these objectives will enable the administration to make informed decisions on safety issues that affect the entire facility. Whereas the safety committee makes recommendations, the administration is responsible for approving recommended policy.

Safety committee members do more than merely attend meetings. To keep the administration abreast of what is going on within the facility, the safety committee receives and reviews incident reports, inspection results, departmental safety policies and procedures, and incident investigation results. After reviewing these documents, the committee then evaluates them and makes suggestions to the administration for action.

The safety committee works closely with the administration to provide the safest possible environment for everyone. The committee accomplishes this objective by providing all new personnel with an orientation to the safety management program. In addition, safety education is provided as part of the continuing education of all personnel. Committee members also serve as safety resources and an advisory group for all employees. The safety committee must also demonstrate evidence that it works with appropriate departments and services to implement committee suggestions. For example, interaction and information exchange with risk management and quality assurance departments are required by the Joint Commission.

For example, the administration is responsible for providing the safety director (or other authorized individual such as the safety officer) with a document that gives him or her the authority to take appropriate action if a life-threatening situation arises or a situation occurs that could cause possible property damage to the facility. This document guarantees the safety director that he or she can take the necessary action without fear of reproach. It was not designed to allow safety directors to take the decision-making process into their own hands, but rather to serve as a means to make decisions in a crisis.

Although the implementation of an effective safety committee is an excellent way to ensure safety in and around the health care facility, there are a number of other safety issues that must be addressed in a variety of different ways.

Fire Safety

Fire safety is a concern that touches every department, with prevention and response being the key ingredients to success. Prevention can be as simple as observing stringent no-smoking rules or as demanding as complying with the life safety management program required by the Joint Commission and meeting the regulations in the Life Safety Code of the National Fire Protection Association (NFPA).

Although a facility's staff may work hard to observe all the necessary safety rules and regulations, fires can happen. A quick response in the event of an emergency can not only save lives, but minimize damage as well. Figure 5-2 lists some departmental responsibilities for planning for and responding to fires. To provide the highest level of fire protection, a master fire plan needs to be in place within the facility, and each employee must know what to do in case of a fire.

Product Liability

In every area of the health care facility, equipment, food, and medication must be kept safe for everyone's use. If a product poses a hazard to patients, employees, or visitors, its use must be discontinued. Health care facilities must take corrective action to protect the safety and well-being of patients, staff, and visitors whenever information on a hazardous product is brought to the facility's attention. (This is a requirement of the U.S. Food and Drug Administration (FDA) and will be discussed in detail in chapter 6.)

When the FDA determines a product to be unsafe, it notifies the facility. It is then the facility's responsibility to take the appropriate action to correct the situation, such as replacing the product. If a facility fails to take action on a recalled product and a serious accident results because the product is still in use, the facility may be held responsible for much of the liability.

Patient Safety

Professional liability risks can have catastrophic effects on the financial well-being of health care facilities. Incidents involving medical–clinical situations are the basis of the most costly claims and suits, so ensuring patient safety is a high priority for health care facilities. By utilizing cost-efficient, integrated approaches to safety, risk management, and quality assurance, facilities can maximize efforts to deliver high-quality patient care and at the same time minimize potential financial loss.

Organizations accredited by the Joint Commission are required to implement the process of *safety management* to study the quality of the patient care environment. Facilities are expected to establish measurable standards of performance and processes designed to ensure that desirable outcomes are achieved and undesirable outcomes are avoided in the application of technology to patients and the patient care environment. This approach encompasses both risk management and quality assurance in addition to safety.

Facilities need to have procedures in place to prevent patient injury. For example, burns can inflict considerable pain and prolong patient stays. Burns are represented to an inordinate degree in patient neglect and medical malpractice suits. Sources of patient burns are scalding water and spills of hot food. Electrical appliances and outlets also create the potential for electrical shock and burns. Figure 5-3 (on p. 68) summarizes safety tips to prevent injuries from electrical appliances and devices.

Ensuring patient safety is oriented toward problem identification, prevention, and resolution. By integrating concepts of overall risk management into safety concepts, facilities can enhance not only the safety program, but employee morale, financial stability, and patient care as well.

Employee Accident Prevention

When administrators consider ways to make their health care facilities safer and more cost-effective, one area that many overlook is worker's compensation. Many on-the-job accidents are caused by unsafe acts rather than unsafe conditions. Some reasons cited

Figure 5-2. Fire Plan Responsibilities for Individual Departments

Nursing Units

Before a fire occurs:

1. One person on the 11 p.m.–7 a.m. shift should be assigned from each patient floor to act as a member of the fire brigade. Another should be assigned to secure a fire extinguisher at his or her location and be ready to respond, if necessary.

2. One person should be designated to turn on all corridor lights.

3. One person should be assigned to monitor the telephone to answer emergency calls or relay messages.

4. One person should be responsible for ensuring that all room doors are closed.

5. A list of patients should be convenient to see that all are accounted for.

6. Every nurse should become familiar with the facility fire plan.

In the event of a fire:

1. Carry out immediate emergency response.

2. Clear exits and elevator area. Do not allow elevators to be used.

3. If fire is in your area, ensure that all oxygen in operation is shut off in a safe manner. Oxygen shut-off valves are located _____. The (title) will make the decision as to when oxygen operation will be shut off.

4. If fire is not in the area, nursing managers should be prepared to use their personnel to care for patients transferred to the area or dispatch personnel to other areas.

5. Reassure patients who may become disturbed by the commotion.

Department Managers

Before a fire occurs:

1. Become familiar with the facility fire plan.

2. See that employees in their departments have been instructed as to their respective duties in case of fire.

In the event of a fire:

1. See that these duties are carried out.

2. Immediately upon hearing the alarm, ensure that all doors and windows in the area are closed.

Plant Services/Maintenance

Before a fire occurs:

1. Become familiar with the facility fire plan.

2. Designate appropriate personnel as members of the fire brigade.

3. Assign one person on the 7 a.m.–3 p.m. shift to meet the fire department at a designated entrance and secure a designated elevator at ground level for their use.

In the event of a fire:

1. Carry out immediate emergency response.

2. The director of maintenance will report to emergency control center, if a member of the emergency control group.

3. Regulate air-handling equipment.

4. Secure electrical room, boiler room, and other maintenance areas, as necessary.

Housekeeping

Before a fire occurs:

1. Become familiar with the facility fire plan.

2. The director of housekeeping will designate appropriate housekeeping personnel as fire brigade members.

Figure 5-2. Continued

In the event of a fire:

1. Carry out immediate emergency response.

2. All other housekeeping personnel remain in their work areas and assist when directed.

3. If necessary, help remove any patient to a safe area.

4. On the 3 p.m.–11 p.m. shift, one person will be assigned to meet the fire department at a designated area and secure a designated elevator for their use.

Dietary

1. Before a fire occurs, become familiar with the facility fire plan.

In the event of a fire:

1. Carry out immediate emergency response.

2. If fire or smoke is in the area, turn off gas and electrical machinery.

3. Personnel are to remain in the department.

4. If necessary, remove any person to a safe area.

5. Await instruction from emergency control center and be prepared to assist wherever needed.

Laundry

1. Before a fire occurs, become familiar with the facility fire plan.

In the event of fire:

1. Carry out immediate emergency response.

2. If fire or smoke is in the area, turn off machines.

3. Personnel are to remain in the department.

4. Await instructions from emergency control center (described in detail in chapter 8), and be prepared to assist wherever needed.

All Other Departments

1. Before a fire occurs, become familiar with the facility fire plan.

In the event of a fire:

1. Carry out immediate emergency response.

2. Personnel are to remain in their departments.

3. If necessary, remove any person to a safe area.

4. Await instructions from emergency control center and be prepared to assist wherever needed.

Source: *Safety Guide for Health Care Institutions*, 4th ed., published by American Hospital Publishing, copyright 1989, pp. 106–107.

for accidents are inadequate training, confusing instructions, fatigue, carelessness, impractical procedures, or complicated safety measures that may cause rather than prevent accidents. Accident prevention is an important goal for its own sake, and it becomes even more important when the cost of accidents is considered.

The high cost of accidents and injuries may not always be evident. There are direct costs such as medical, hospital, rehabilitation expenses, and worker's compensation payments. However, many less-obvious indirect costs are generally not covered by insurance, such as lost efficiency, the cost of investigating the accident, report time, replacing the worker, and tool and equipment damage. As accidents and claims increase, so do insurance premiums. If claims become a serious problem, the facility could lose its insurability.

If a facility continually looks to the insurance company to pay its high cost of claims, premiums rise and profits shrink. In addition, if the administration repeatedly relies on

Figure 5-3. Electrical Appliance Safety Measures

Heating pads and hot-water bottles

- Never place a heating pad or hot-water bottle directly against an unconscious person, a person in shock, an infant, or a dressing.
- Check the temperature of pads and bottles. Temperatures should never exceed 130° F (54.4° C) for adults and 120° F (48.8° C) for children.
- Check skin temperature shortly after applying a pad or bottle. Do not accept the patient's opinion on his or her comfort.
- Check soundness of each item before use. Heating pads are electrical appliances and subject to all regulations set for electrical equipment.
- Use tape, binders, or straps to keep units in place. Do not use pins or clamps.
- Use heating pad only on low setting.

Infrared lamps and light cradles

- Use infrared lamps and light cradles only on the physician's orders.
- If the site to be treated is near the head, protect the patient's eyes with a towel or washcloth.
- Place the equipment at least 18 inches from the patient's body. In a light cradle only a 25-watt bulb is used.
- Ensure that equipment has guards.
- Attend the patient the entire time the equipment is in use. The attendant must be a staff member, not a visitor.
- Inspect wiring and connections daily.

Steam inhalators

- Inspect the steam inhalator equipment before using it to be sure it is filled with water.
- Prevent hot vapor from concentrating on the patient's body.
- Make sure the equipment does not overheat.
- Do not place steam inhalators on bedside tables where patients may accidentally knock them over.

All burns require immediate attention and notification of the patient's physician.

Personal electrical appliances

- Use of personal electrical appliances should be limited.
- Elderly persons, children, and patients with psychiatric conditions should be closely supervised while using personal electrical appliances.
- Check these appliances when they are brought in and, for long-term care residents, regularly thereafter for worn wiring, connections, and plugs.

Source: *Safety Guide for Health Care Institutions*, 4th ed., published by American Hospital Publishing, copyright 1989, p. 71.

the facility's insurance to pay the cost of an accident or injury, it is making an uninformed decision because generally, only a portion of the actual claim cost is covered by insurance.

Here again, prevention is the key. Ongoing training for all employees reinforces the importance of reducing incidents. By implementing effective accident prevention and comprehensive safety programs, the high cost of providing worker's compensation can be reduced.

Preemployment Screening

Encouraging the personnel department to hire safety-conscious individuals is another step the administration can take in the overall safety program. Because employee safety begins during the hiring process, strong consideration should be given to the applicant's skills, experience, and any physical limitations prior to job placement. A preemployment physical and a medical history questionnaire are also good tools for determining physical suitability for a job. An employer can opt to require physical examinations, although specific guidelines must be followed. Obtaining information about the employee's past medical history should be done in accordance with state and federal guidelines.

Emergency Preparedness

Another area of safety that necessitates the administration's active participation is emergency preparedness. In the event of a disaster, the community looks to the health care facility for assistance. The facility must respond to an emergency situation by continuing to serve the community with as few interruptions to service as possible.

The most effective way to achieve this goal is through comprehensive, coordinated planning with staff members and appropriate community agencies. A carefully prepared and successfully implemented disaster plan is key to saving lives.

The Joint Commission requires specific plans for evacuations; fires; bombs; interruption of electrical, gas, and water services; and other emergencies. (Figure 5-4 lists some possible disasters that could affect health care delivery.)

Hazard Communication

Before hazardous materials enter a facility, a comprehensive hazardous materials plan should be in place. The plan records what chemicals are being used in which department, along with their hazards and other pertinent information. Most important, part of the plan is to train employees in the proper ways to handle the harmful materials in order to reduce risk to their safety and health.

Another aspect of hazard communication involves a facility's disclosure of the hazardous chemicals that its workers are exposed to. The 1983 Hazard Communication Standard published by OSHA proposed that a worker has a *right to know* (a term that soon identified the standard) what chemicals he or she handles or works around. (This law is covered in chapter 6 under OSHA.)

The Occupational Safety and Health Administration can exact penalties and fines for failure to comply with the right-to-know law. However, along with protection from regulatory censure, implementing a hazard communication program also lays down a strong foundation for hazardous waste management and other precautions. Material safety data sheets (MSDSs) and lists will allow for easier tracking of chemicals when they become wastes, and employees will already be trained in where to go for information and how to protect themselves.

Figure 5-4. Potential Disasters That Could Affect Health Care Delivery

- Train accident
- Epidemic of food poisoning or other illness
- Nuclear accident
- Internal fire
- Fire in the community
- Chemical spill or release
- Airplane crash
- Multiple-car collision
- School bus wreck
- Bomb threat
- Terrorist attack
- Hostage situation
- Strikes, picketing, protests
- Power outage
- Utility (water, heat, natural gas) failure
- Computer failure
- Earthquake
- Monsoon
- Hurricane
- Tornado
- Blizzard
- Snowstorm
- Thunderstorm
- Drought
- Natural gas leak
- Building collapse
- Industrial or construction accident
- VIP disaster (for example, assassination or illness of a public figure)
- Flood

Source: *Safety Guide for Health Care Institutions*, 4th ed., published by American Hospital Publishing, copyright 1989, p. 121.

Medical Waste and Hazardous Materials

One of the biggest challenges facing administrators today is minimizing the environmental and economic effects of medical waste and hazardous materials. Understanding the difference between the two and becoming sensitized to the issues surrounding them are important.

After their use, hazardous chemicals become hazardous waste. However, although they are wastes, the materials still pose risks to the facility and the environment. They must be contained appropriately and stored under proper conditions. Most important, facilities cannot dispose of these wastes in a haphazard manner. Improper disposal can pollute the environment and endanger the life and health of people and wildlife in the community.

Therefore, *hazardous waste* can be defined as chemical waste that poses long-term risks to the environment. An example of this would be a hospital pouring a known hazardous chemical, such as mercury, down the drain. Mercury is EP (extraction procedure) toxic and may release toxic substances into the groundwater or cause a poison hazard to human health or the environment. Even though this might be done only drops at a time, it nonetheless creates an environmental threat.

Medical waste includes two definitions: infectious waste and regulated medical waste. *Infectious waste* is waste that is capable of transmitting or producing disease. Examples of infectious waste are contaminated sharps, human blood and blood products, pathological waste (body parts and tissues), and laboratory waste.

Medical waste includes both infectious waste as well as other waste that, although it may not be infectious, may be offensive to the public. An example of this would be contaminated waste such as IV tubing or used bandages washing ashore. This type of waste not only presents a potential health and safety threat to citizens in the community, but also creates an eyesore.

Added to the confusion of clearly defining medical waste and hazardous materials is that the terms are often used interchangeably. Local, state, and federal governments may also define them differently. For the most part, hazardous waste poses long-term risks to the environment, whereas infectious waste poses short-lived risks.

Learning how to manage hazardous substances from the time they enter the facility until their final disposal is a vital link in the safety process. Health care facilities are being increasingly regulated on hazardous/infectious materials by numerous governmental agencies, and the results of their findings are reported in newspapers and on television.

Instead of dodging the public's concern regarding this issue, health care facilities need to be aware that effective communication within the facility as well as in the community is part of the total medical waste and hazardous materials management process.

There are several ways a facility can work to ensure safe use and disposal of these potentially hazardous materials. For example, developing a comprehensive program that records and monitors chemicals as they enter the facility, tracks where they are dispensed, and includes the necessary precautions to protect employees as they use and work around these hazardous materials is very effective.

Another alternative is substitution. Increasingly, manufacturers are producing non-hazardous (or less-hazardous) substitutes for products that previously contained hazardous chemicals. Department heads can contact the manufacturers or distributors of chemicals or chemical compounds that create hazardous by-products to see whether they have nonhazardous or less-hazardous equivalents. The number of possible substitutions may be surprising. Even if they are more expensive, the cost will probably be made up in savings on waste storage, treatment, and disposal.

Developing an emergency plan in case of an accident or a spill is another way a facility can promote safety. By doing this, the administration is not only making the facility a safer place to work, but it is helping to protect the community from a hazardous materials disaster as well.

☐ Equipment and Technology

Just as medical advancements have had an enormous impact on patient care, so has technology in the field of safety. No longer are fire extinguishers or safety glasses the only items that fall under the heading of safety equipment.

Although fire extinguishers and safety glasses do play an important part in safety, the list of safety equipment now includes a number of other items. Here is a brief description of the safety equipment and technology that normally fall under the safety department's jurisdiction:

- *Emergency chemical decontamination:* This is done to decontaminate emergency room patients exposed to potentially deadly chemicals. The location should have access to a water supply, protective clothing, a self-contained breathing apparatus, and detergents. The location should also have a self-contained vent system. Contaminated liquids and solid wastes must be disposed of according to federal, state, and local hazardous waste regulations.
- *Fire extinguishers:* Facilities must provide appropriate fire extinguishers for the type of fire that is likely to occur in that area.
- *Personal protective equipment:* Although the safety director is not directly responsible for keeping these items in stock, he or she should be available to help decide when to use personal protective equipment and what type to purchase for employee use. For example:
  - Gloves (for handling chemicals and hot, wet, or sharp objects)
  - Eye and face protection (against chips, sparks, glass, and splashes)
  - Hearing protection (against noise)
  - Respirators and self-contained breathing apparatuses (SCBAs) (against gases, vapors, asbestos, and so forth)
- *Protective equipment for working with radioactive materials:* This includes mechanical pipetting devices, lead aprons, and goggles.
- *Engineering controls:* These are pieces of equipment or techniques that reduce employee exposure. For asbestos they include ventilation systems, local exhaust systems, or the wetting of asbestos-containing materials to keep fibers from becoming airborne.
- *Container labeling:* All chemicals in the health care facility must be labeled with the identity of the chemical and proper health warnings.
- *Technology and equipment for cleaning up hazardous material spills:* For example, the laboratory would use a spill cleanup kit containing:
  - Spill absorbent
  - Neutralizer for acids
  - Neutralizer for alkalis
  - Neutralizer for mercury
  - Pan, gloves, brush, and apron
- *MSDSs:* These are technical documents containing detailed information on hazardous chemicals.
- *Protective barrier shields:* These are used when opening stoppered tubes in the laboratory and performing work that may cause splashing.
- *Eyewash station:* This is used if an eye is splashed.
- *Emergency safety shower:* This is used for a major spill involving areas of the body other than the eyes.
- *Industrial hygiene:* This involves recognizing, evaluating, and controlling environmental conditions that may have adverse effects on health, may be uncomfortable or irritating, or may have some undesired effect on the ability of individuals to perform their normal work. This is an employee monitoring process that recognizes problems such as dust, vapors, heat stress, or repetitive motion.

☐ Safety and Compliance

Through the development of advanced medicines and equipment modern technology has saved millions of lives, but in doing so it has created an abundance of unique problems as well. Coming to grips with the risks involved and making the health care facility a safer place for everyone have involved the formation of a number of regulatory agencies. These organizations can be divided into two principal types, governmental and voluntary, and are described in chapter 6.

Governmental compliance agencies do everything from establishing regulations and enforcing them to publishing information and operating offices that provide assistance in understanding the regulations. In addition to state and local agencies, several governmental bodies work together to regulate safety within the health care facility.

☐ Program Evaluation

Is safety working within the health care facility? The answer to this question may be another question: Is safety *not* working? There are several indicators that may help answer these questions: Are insurance premiums skyrocketing? Are incidents more frequent? Are employees unhappy with their working conditions? Taking time to find the answers to these and other pressing questions will not only create a safer facility, but will save dollars in the long run.

Knowing a safety problem exists is not enough. To help ensure the highest standards of patient care, health care facilities should conduct ongoing safety assessments designed to provide specific information that will reduce liability, prevent accidents, build employee morale, and improve the overall operation of the facility.

Assessments should be done at least annually for areas that are not directly involved in patient care and semiannually for those areas that are. The assessment team should include the safety director and representatives from administration, management, and employees. In each department, the assessment team will work closely with the department head who, for that part of the survey, becomes a temporary member of the team.

The safety assessment should be developed through the safety committee. To ensure that employees have input, the first step may be to mail questionnaires to department heads or talk with key personnel. After this step of the assessment is complete, a walk-through of the facility should be conducted to identify visible areas of risk. Checklists are useful when conducting visual inspections (figure 5-5). In addition, reports and records should be reviewed to help identify existing practices and programs and their perceived effectiveness (figure 5-6, p. 74). These are important steps in building a team effort for problem solving.

The final steps in the safety assessment are ongoing evaluations and follow-up reports. These reports define existing programs that are working for the facility, identify problems, and make recommendations for prioritizing program development. The results of the safety assessment should be shared with the administration, board of directors, medical staff, and employees. The various factions of the facility can then work together to make the necessary changes and improvements.

As the safety assessment process uncovers potential threats and vulnerabilities, the administration can use the information as a valuable tool to enhance the facility's operation.

☐ Summary

Safety plays an important role in the daily operation of any health care facility. Effective safety management not only assures employees that they have a safe working environment,

Figure 5-5. Safety Inspection Checklist for Storerooms

Item	Yes	No	Comments on Deficiencies Noted and Action Required	Date Corrected
Are storerooms well lighted?				
Are storerooms orderly?				
Are exits and aisles of storerooms clear at all times?				
Are rubbish, empty cartons, and paper disposed of immediately?				
Are heavy items always stored on the lower shelves?				
Are spillage items always stored below eye level?				
Are objects that might roll blocked?				
Are materials stored clear of sprinkler heads (at least 18 inches) and other fire-fighting equipment?				
When cases are stacked head high or higher, are the cases crisscrossed to eliminate danger of falling cases?				
Are flammable liquids: Stored in approved containers?				
Stored in safe quantities?				
Stored in approved cabinets?				
Are storage shelves adequate for the weight involved?				
Are stepladders, rather than "make-shifts," always used to stand on?				
Are all stepladders in safe condition?				
Do portable ladders have safety feet?				
Are employees lifting heavy objects in the proper way?				
Are corrugated cartons opened with a sharp knife or special cutting tool, rather than pried loose with the hand or fingers?				

Source: Adapted, with permission, from National Safety Council. *Long Term Care Safety Management Manual: A Handbook for Practical Application.* Chicago: National Safety Council, 1987, pp. 135–65.

Figure 5-6. Information to Review When Conducting a Safety Assessment

- Employee incident reports
- Safety committee minutes
- Patient and employee safety policies
- Selected job descriptions

- Joint Commission survey report (current)
- Fire marshal report (current)
- Insurance company loss control reports (two each for professional liability and worker's compensation)

but also allows patients to enjoy an atmosphere that is free from unnecessary risks and hazards.

Having an effective safety program that addresses pertinent safety issues within the facility, as well as within the community, will give the administration confidence that the facility is delivering the highest quality of patient care.

☐ References and Bibliography

Chaff, L. F. *Building a Successful Safety Committee.* Chattanooga, TN: Chaff & Company, 1990.

Chaff, L. F. *Managing Health Care Hazards.* Chicago: Labelmaster, 1988.

Chaff, L. F. *Safety Guide for Health Care Institutions.* 4th ed. Chicago: American Hospital Publishing, 1989.

Joint Commission on Accreditation of Healthcare Organizations. Plant, technology and safety management. *Accreditation Manual for Hospitals.* Oakbrook Terrace, IL: JCAHO, 1991, P.L. 199–208.

Lee, L. *Safety Management for Health Care Facilities.* Chicago: American Hospital Association, 1989.

National Safety Council. *Health Care Section Safety Survey.* Chicago: NSC, July 1990.

U.S. Department of Health and Human Services. *Guidelines for Protecting the Safety and Health of Health Care Workers.* Washington, DC: U.S. Government Printing Office, Sept. 1988.

Chapter 6

Codes, Standards, and Regulation Compliance

Douglas S. Erickson

□ Overview

During the past century, the United States has seen the most explosive growth in the medical field that has ever been witnessed throughout history. Not only can people's brains be scanned to detect tumors and other growths, but thanks to the advancements in modern technology, treatments have been developed that can cure an almost infinite number of illnesses and diseases.

Modern technology has saved millions of lives, but not without a price tag. Wonder drugs often have serious side effects. Complicated machinery not only malfunctions, but can create possible electrical and fire hazards as well. Substances that make treatment easier or more successful, such as anesthesia gases and radioactive materials, may at the same time pose hazards to employees and the environment. Even the routine management of health care facilities is not without its share of problems. Wet or slippery floors can cause accidents; blocked fire exits pose serious safety problems.

Getting the situation under control and creating a safe environment for patients, guests, and employees are tremendous tasks. To help staff in health care facilities understand the magnitude of the potential problems they face every day and find solutions to these problems, a number of regulatory agencies and organizations have been established.

These organizations can be divided into two principal types—governmental and voluntary. The following sections define the two types and describe the activities and responsibilities of major organizations within each group.

□ Governmental Compliance Agencies

Governmental compliance agencies are those organizations that the government—federal, state, or local—has endowed with the authority to establish regulations and enforce them. Many times, the rules these agencies promulgate have the force of law, and violators

Parts of this chapter were reprinted, with permission, from *Safety Guide for Health Care Institutions,* 4th ed., published by American Hospital Publishing, Inc., copyright 1989.

may be subject to civil and even criminal penalties. Other times, they may publish only guidelines, but still base their inspections and citations on these recommendations.

In all cases, these agencies publish information and operate offices that concerned individuals can contact for answers or assistance. As government entities, such agencies are public servants, but all too often employers fail to make use of these resources. These agencies are often happy to help health care facilities with any concerns they may have; if they cannot, at the very least they will usually make a referral to an organization that can assist. For this reason, information on how to contact each agency is listed in appendix C.

Occupational Safety and Health Administration

In 1970, during the Nixon administration, Congress passed the Occupational Safety and Health Act. This act created an agency that would be controlled by the Department of Labor and would require employers to ensure safe and healthful working conditions for employees in the workplace. The act gave every employee the right to a reasonably secure, risk-free environment that the employer must maintain. The agency created by this act was called the Occupational Safety and Health Administration (OSHA).

Soon after its birth, OSHA began to develop regulations for employers that governed workplace safety. The agency summarized the responsibility of employers in its General Duty Clause, namely that the employer must provide "employment and a place of employment which are free from recognized hazards that are causing or are likely to cause death or serious physical harm" to employees.

On the basis of this foundation, OSHA moved on to write other standards on more specific safety issues for various industries. Once these requirements were established, it became the task of all employers and employees to familiarize themselves with the standards that apply to them and to comply conscientiously with these regulations at all times.

The Occupational Safety and Health Administration has issued numerous regulations that affect health care facilities, especially on general safety. For example, there are OSHA rules covering the use of ladders and scaffolds, the condition of exits, electrical safety, lifting techniques, and the use of personal protective equipment. Moreover, the Joint Commission on Accreditation of Healthcare Organizations (Joint Commission) requires compliance with basic OSHA safety regulations.

Other areas of OSHA regulation and guidance for health care facilities include the storage and transportation of compressed gas cylinders, the control of waste anesthetic gas, the handling of cytotoxic (antineoplastic) drugs, and the use of X-ray equipment. In addition, OSHA is utilizing enforceable guidelines for protecting workers from occupational exposure to AIDS, hepatitis B, and other blood-borne diseases. These guidelines (29 C.F.R. 1910.1030) are expected to become a final rule in 1991.

Finally, although this is by no means an exhaustive list, OSHA oversees compliance with its Hazard Communication Standard. First published in 1983, this standard gives employees the right to know what hazardous chemicals they work with. Although the rule at first only applied to manufacturing industries, in 1987 it was expanded to cover all employers, including health care facilities. Under the "right-to-know" standard, as it came to be called, all employees must be informed about the chemicals they work with, the chemicals' hazards, and how to protect themselves. The Hazard Communication Standard has a number of specific requirements for employers, including a written program and training for employees.

The Occupational Safety and Health Administration enforces its requirements through workplace inspections. These can occur for five reasons:

- Imminent danger
- Catastrophes or fatal accidents

- Employee complaints
- Programmed inspections for high-hazard industries
- Follow-up inspections

Inspections are conducted to determine whether any safety and health hazards have been overlooked by the employer and, when necessary, citations are issued and fines levied.

If the potential harm represents an immediate threat to the health or life of employees, OSHA will take immediate steps to remove the hazard. Otherwise, OSHA may issue a citation that may still result in penalties or civil or criminal fines. However, OSHA assures employers that consideration is given to the appropriateness of the penalty, the severity of the violation, the size of the facility, the good faith of the employer, and the record of previous violations.

Many resources exist to help staff and supervisors understand what OSHA expects from them. This awareness is intrinsic to an effective safety program, because OSHA was established to ensure workplace safety. In many ways, OSHA standards and guidelines relate directly to the health care facility. Understanding them can greatly enhance safety and the smooth operation of the facility. For more information, contact your OSHA regional office (see table 6-1) or call or write to the federal office.

U.S. Environmental Protection Agency

The Environmental Protection Agency (EPA) exercises control over the release of harmful materials into the environment. As with OSHA, the EPA has written both regulations and general guidelines. These rules and recommendations define which substances can be hazardous to human health and the environment, outline formal procedures for handling these materials, govern the operation of waste disposal sites, and establish a system for dealing with environmental accidents such as leaks or spills.

As patient care becomes more and more complex, health care facilities increasingly rely on hazardous chemicals during routine operation. Whereas OSHA's Hazard Communication Standard covers the use of these substances by employees in the performance of their jobs, EPA rules apply primarily to the effects of the materials on the environment. The EPA's purview also extends to infectious wastes because they, too, possess a potential to endanger humans and the environment, although the degree of possible harm remains a matter of debate. In order to effect a comprehensive system of control for dangerous wastes, the EPA has published numerous rules and guidelines. The following have the greatest effect on health care:

- *Clean Air Act:* In 1970, Congress passed this act to empower the EPA to set permissible levels for the emission of hazardous substances into the air. Congress strengthened this act by passing revisions in 1990.
- *Clean Water Act:* In an effort to buttress the 1972 Federal Water Pollution Control Act, the Clean Water Act was passed in 1977. This act limits the discharge of hazardous substances into our waterways. The act established the National Pollutant Discharge Elimination System (NPDES), which requires permits for the discharge of harmful materials into water. In 1987, this act was bolstered by a congressional reauthorization.
- *Toxic Substances Control Act (TSCA) of 1976:* This legislation regulates the manufacture, distribution, and use of toxic chemicals. It requires manufacturers to notify the EPA when proposing new chemicals and regularly assesses existing hazardous chemicals. The TSCA may limit or prohibit the use of some chemicals, and this may have an impact on health care. For example, the use of polychlorinated biphenyls (PCBs), except in a totally enclosed system, has been disallowed. The transformers and capacitors in some older facilities may contain PCBs and may not always be regarded as being in a totally enclosed system.

Table 6-1. OSHA Regional Offices

Region	Geographical Area Covered	OSHA Regional Office
I	Connecticut,* Maine, Massachusetts, New Hampshire, Rhode Island, Vermont*	16-18 North Street 1 Dock Square Building 4th Floor Boston, MA 02109 Telephone: 617/565-1161
II	New Jersey, New York,* Puerto Rico	201 Varick Street 6th Floor New York, NY 10014 Telephone: 212/337-2325
III	Delaware, District of Columbia, Maryland,* Pennsylvania, Virginia,* West Virginia	Gateway Building, Suite 2100 3535 Market Street Philadelphia, PA 19104 Telephone: 215/596-1201
IV	Alabama, Florida, Georgia, Kentucky,* Mississippi, North Carolina,* South Carolina,* Tennessee*	1375 Peachtree Street, N.E. Suite 587 Atlanta, GA 30367 Telephone: 404/347-3573
V	Illinois, Indiana,* Michigan,* Minnesota,* Ohio, Wisconsin	230 South Dearborn Street 32nd Floor, Room 3244 Chicago, IL 60604 Telephone: 312/353-2200
VI	Arkansas, Louisiana, New Mexico,* Oklahoma, Texas	525 Griffin Street Room 602 Dallas, TX 75202 Telephone: 214/767-3731
VII	Iowa,* Kansas, Missouri, Nebraska	911 Walnut Street, Room 406 Kansas City, MO 64106 Telephone: 816/374-5861
VIII	Colorado, Montana, North Dakota, South Dakota, Utah,* Wyoming*	Federal Building, Room 1576 1961 Stout Street Denver, CO 80294 Telephone: 303/844-3061
IX	Arizona,* California,* Hawaii,* Nevada*	71 Stevenson Street 4th Floor San Francisco, CA 94105 Telephone: 415/995-5672
X	Alaska,* Idaho,* Oregon,* Washington*	Federal Office Building Room 6003 909 First Avenue Seattle, WA 98174 Telephone: 206/442-5930

Source: *Safety Guide for Health Care Institutions,* 4th ed., published by American Hospital Publishing, Inc., copyright 1989, p. 22.

*These states and territories operate their own OSHA-approved job safety and health programs (except Connecticut and New York, whose plans cover public employees only).

- *Resource Conservation and Recovery Act (RCRA) of 1976:* This is the act that has the greatest impact on health care facilities and other waste generators. It establishes a system for the control of hazardous wastes from the time they are generated until their final disposal, from "cradle to grave." The RCRA divides waste generators into categories based on the amount of waste generated; requires permits for generators, transporters, and disposal facilities; and sets up a manifesting system whereby wastes are tracked from generation to disposal.

—*Comprehensive Environmental Response, Compensation, and Liability Act (CERCLA) of 1980:* Called Superfund, this act allocates funding and direction for the cleanup of contaminated waste sites. It also confers liability on all involved with the waste site, even if they did not directly cause the contamination. Under CERCLA, hospitals have had to help pay for the cleanup of waste sites to which they have sent their wastes.

—*The Superfund Amendments and Reauthorization Act (SARA) of 1986:* This act reauthorizes and strengthens CERCLA. In addition, Title III of SARA establishes a system of response in the event of an environmental disaster. Title III gives some hospitals additional environmental responsibilities. It requires hospitals to coordinate environmental safety plans with community agencies.

- *Infectious Waste Guidelines:* In 1986, the EPA published guidelines for the handling, treatment, and disposal of infectious waste. These are guidelines and do not possess the force of law. However, because of well-publicized medical waste dumpings and societal concerns, the EPA has announced it will reconsider its policy of just publishing guidelines on this subject.

Taken together, these EPA rules and guidelines represent a broad base of responsibility for health care facilities. The laws empowering the EPA are summarized in figure 6-1. In addition, regulations are expanding and changing almost daily, as is evident from the rules that have been strengthened, reauthorized, or reconsidered. Compounding the problem, individual citizens may sue for damage that results from the release of a hazardous substance.

Thus administrators and personnel should be aware that the EPA is a major source of regulatory control for them. However, the EPA can also act as an excellent source of guidance and information. It publishes informative guides to help facilities understand and comply with regulations, such as its 1986 *Understanding the Small Quantity Generator Hazardous Waste Rules: A Handbook for Small Businesses* and *EPA Guide for Infectious Waste Management.* Table 6-2 lists the EPA regional offices.

Centers for Disease Control

The Centers for Disease Control (CDC) safeguards the health of the American people by controlling and preventing disease. It conducts research and publishes results, often

Figure 6-1. Laws Empowering the EPA

Law	Allows EPA to:
1. Clean Air Act, 1970	Set permissible levels for hazardous and visible emissions into the air.
2. Clean Water Act, 1977 (reauthorized 1987)	Limit discharge of pollutants into waterways. Set up the NPDES.
3. Toxic Substances Control Act, 1976	Regulate manufacture, distribution, and use of toxic chemicals.
4. Resource Conservation and Recovery Act, 1976	Establish system by which wastes are tracked from "cradle to grave."
5. Comprehensive Environmental Response, Compensation, and Liability Act, 1980 (also known as Superfund)	Set aside funds for cleanup of contaminated waste sites. Broaden liability for contaminated sites.
6. Superfund Amendments and Reauthorization Act, 1986	Reauthorize CERCLA. Establish system of response for environmental disasters.

Source: *Safety Guide for Health Care Institutions,* 4th ed., published by American Hospital Publishing, Inc., copyright 1989, p. 23.

Note: NPDES = National Pollutant Discharge Elimination System.

Table 6-2. EPA Regional Offices

Region	Geographical Area Covered	U.S. EPA Regional Office
I	Connecticut, Maine, Massachusetts, New Hampshire, Rhode Island, Vermont	State Waste Programs Branch JFK Federal Building Boston, MA 02203
II	New Jersey, New York, Puerto Rico, Virgin Islands	Air and Waste Management Division 26 Federal Plaza New York, NY 10278
III	Delaware, District of Columbia, Maryland, Pennsylvania, Virginia, West Virginia	Waste Management Branch MS 3HW 34 841 Chestnut Street Philadelphia, PA 19107
IV	Alabama, Florida, Georgia, Kentucky, Mississippi, North Carolina, South Carolina, Tennessee	Hazardous Waste Management Division 345 Courtland Street, N.E. Atlanta, GA 30365
V	Illinois, Indiana, Michigan, Minnesota, Ohio, Wisconsin	RCRA Activities Waste Management Division P.O. Box A3587 Chicago, IL 60690
VI	Arkansas, Louisiana, New Mexico, Oklahoma, Texas	Air and Hazardous Materials Division 1201 Elm Street Inter-First Two Building Dallas, TX 75270
VII	Iowa, Kansas, Missouri, Nebraska	RCRA Branch 726 Minnesota Avenue Kansas City, KS 66620
VIII	Colorado, Montana, North Dakota, South Dakota, Utah, Wyoming	Waste Management Division (8 HWM-ON) One Denver Place, Suite 1300 999 18th Street Denver, CO 80202-2413
IX	Arizona, California, Hawaii, Nevada, American Samoa, Guam	Toxics and Waste Management Division 215 Fremont Street San Francisco, CA 94105
X	Alaska, Idaho, Oregon, Washington	Waste Management Branch—MS-530 1200 Sixth Avenue Seattle, WA 98101

Source: *Safety Guide for Health Care Institutions*, 4th ed., published by American Hospital Publishing, Inc., copyright 1989, p. 24.

in the *Morbidity and Mortality Weekly Report.* This periodical is an up-to-date and thorough reference for health care facilities that want to stay ahead of new guidelines and regulations on such topics as infection control, infectious waste, and worker protection from blood-borne infectious diseases such as AIDS and viruses such as hepatitis B. Various agencies, such as OSHA, the EPA, and the Joint Commission, rely on CDC research and guidelines.

The CDC has six operational units:

- *The Center for Environmental Health* works to control environmentally related and chronic diseases.
- *The Center for Health Promotion and Education* responds to the growing need for disease prevention and promotion of good health.
- *The Center for Prevention Services* cooperates with state and local health agencies on preventive health services.

- *The National Institute for Occupational Safety and Health (NIOSH)* recommends occupational safety and health standards and provides research, training, and technical assistance to promote healthful working conditions. The Occupational Safety and Health Administration relies heavily on NIOSH research in writing new regulations. The NIOSH can be an excellent resource for the employee accident prevention element of safety.
- *The Center for Professional Development and Training* coordinates training to build a national work force committed to disease prevention and control. This is another resource for facilities.
- *The Center for Infectious Diseases* coordinates a national program to investigate, prevent, and control infectious disease. This is where CDC infection control guidelines originate.

Through these six centers, the CDC provides a wide variety of technical information and support services. Health care facilities should avail themselves of the CDC's numerous resources.

U.S. Food and Drug Administration

The Food and Drug Administration (FDA) is charged with supervising the development, testing, and monitoring of food and drug products and medical equipment. The FDA requires the health care facility to take corrective action to protect the safety and well-being of patients, staff, and visitors whenever information on a hazardous product is brought to the facility's attention. It is the responsibility of the facility to obtain, evaluate, and act upon all information concerning hazards of the equipment, food, and medication it uses.

Until the mid-1970s, the FDA had no well-defined control over medical devices. However, in 1976, the Medical Device Amendments to the Federal Food, Drug, and Cosmetics Act (which established the FDA) set up an FDA Bureau of Medical Devices (BMD). The BMD is now called the Center for Devices and Radiological Health, and it possesses the authority to ban or recall products that present a substantial and unreasonable risk for harm. The severity of the hazard determines whether the product is removed from the marketplace. Even the risk is not severe enough to recall the product, the manufacturer still must notify users of the hazard(s).

Depending on the situation, products are recalled through letters, postcards, and telegrams. The FDA may require the manufacturer to send a return-receipt letter to the facility. This document, when signed by an authorized employee of the facility, officially acknowledges that the facility has received the recall notice. It then becomes the facility's responsibility to initiate an organized procedure to communicate the necessary information to all appropriate staff and make arrangements to replace the product, if necessary. If the facility does not take some measures and the recalled product causes a serious accident, much of the liability may be transferred to the facility.

The FDA has also established the Medical Device and Laboratory Product Problem Reporting Program, whereby health care workers can report problems in products they use. This program is geared toward improving communication of hazards resulting from medical products. For further information, contact the Practicioner Reporting System.

Other sources of information on food, drug, or medical device hazards include the *FDA Enforcement Report*, available from the Press Office, Food and Drug Administration, and the *Health Device Alerts*, available from the Emergency Care Research Institute.

U.S. Nuclear Regulatory Commission

The Nuclear Regulatory Commission (NRC) oversees the operation of nuclear power facilities and regulates the handling, use, and disposal of radiological materials. Hospitals may use radiological substances in several areas of operation including nuclear medicine, radiology, clinical laboratories, and research laboratories. The types of materials used in hospitals usually result in low-level radioactive waste.

Radioactive waste is unlike infectious and hazardous waste in that the hazardousness of this waste can only be completely removed by time. That is, over time, radioactive materials decay and become less dangerous. Some hospital radiologicals decay within days. However, for others, the rate of radioactive decay, called the *half-life*, can be very slow; some require thousands of years to become thoroughly harmless. Meanwhile, these substances emit dangerous radiation, which has been associated with cancers, birth defects, and other health problems.

As a result, these materials must be carefully handled during use and adequately contained for disposal. Hazardousness and half-lives vary widely among radiological materials, as do disposal techniques. Contaminated materials may be incinerated, put in landfills, allowed to decay in storage, or disposed of through the sanitary sewer, depending on their type and the applicable regulations. The NRC has published regulations governing these practices in its *Standards for Protection Against Radiation.*

State Requirements

Individual states have requirements for health care facilities on many of the same topics as federal agency regulations. However, the state requirements may be more rigorous or extensive than federal standards. These state rules are usually enforced through licensure or the periodic inspection and relicensure process. States may legislate practices in many areas, including:

- *Occupational safety and health:* Federal OSHA gives states the option of implementing their own workplace safety and health programs rather than adopting the federal program. These state OSHA programs must be at least as stringent as the federal program.
- *Hazardous waste:* States may establish their own EPA hazardous waste management agencies to assist in compliance with EPA rules and possibly expand on them.
- *Infectious waste:* Although this is rapidly changing, the greatest source of rule making for infectious waste is state agencies. Regulations are usually issued by the board of health or state EPA, if there is one. In addition, local sewer districts may have rules for the disposal of hazardous or infectious materials through the sewer.
- *Worker's compensation:* A common denominator for all states is the existence of worker's compensation laws, which are generally enforced by the state's attorney general or similar agent. The penalties for failure to comply with these laws, as well as the actual compensation to injured employees, are cumulative and can cause financial hardship for any size facility. Effective accident prevention and comprehensive safety programs can minimize unreasonable worker's compensation costs.
- *Fire and health codes:* The state or local fire authority, normally the fire marshal's office, verifies that fire safety requirements are met by using its own state codes and National Fire Protection Association (NFPA) codes (which are voluntary codes). In addition, health or fire department officials, or the authority having jurisdiction, will verify compliance with required infection control techniques, sanitation practices, proper storage and disposal of hazardous materials, and training of staff in the proper identification and control of hazardous substances.

Because state and local requirements on these and other subjects may differ from or expand upon national standards, it is crucial that health care facilities gain an awareness of the regulations in their area that affect them. As with federal mandates, facilities should be aware that regional requirements may change as new information becomes available. Abiding by state and local rules can provide a strong foundation for compliance with federal and voluntary standards.

Building Codes

To ensure that safety standards are followed when new buildings are constructed or existing ones are repaired, building codes have been established. The codes may be adapted either at the local or state level and are enforced by a building official.

The typical building code applies to the construction, alteration, addition, repair, removal, demolition, use, location, occupancy, and maintenance of all buildings and structures. Three model building codes have been developed and are used within the United States. These codes and the organizations that publish them are as follows:

- *BOCA National Building Code:* Building Officials and Code Administrators International, Inc.
- *Standard Building Code:* Southern Building Code Congress International, Inc.
- *Uniform Building Code:* The International Conference of Building Officials

Each of these groups also publishes companion codes, such as mechanical, plumbing, and gas codes, which may apply to construction projects. The staff of each organization is available to provide interpretations of the various codes for members. Educational programs, monthly publications, technical documents, and annual conferences that include continuing education opportunities related to code issues are also provided by these organizations.

Some jurisdictions may choose to write their own codes in lieu of adopting one of the model codes. It is not mandatory for the codes to follow established building codes.

In addition to these codes and standards, many health departments have promulgated regulations on constructing and equipping medical facilities. These standards typically address functional program requirements and may also include references to building codes or NFPA 101. Many states reference a Public Health Service document entitled *Guidelines for Construction and Equipment of Hospital and Medical Facilities.*

□ Voluntary Compliance Organizations

Just as not-for-profit health care facilities have always, in a way, "volunteered" medical services to the community, so have voluntary organizations set standards for the health care industry. These organizations and their standards are highly regarded, and their accreditation of a facility is often evidence that the facility places high priority on safety and health.

Voluntary organizations act out of a sincere desire to enhance patient care and ensure that the facility is a safe environment for its inhabitants. Moreover, many governmental agencies look to these voluntary groups for technical assistance in developing regulations for the health care industry. When incorporated into federal, state, or local regulations, voluntary standards become compulsory.

The NFPA, the Joint Commission, the American National Standards Institute, and the Compressed Gas Association represent just a few of the myriad helpful voluntary organizations that are too numerous to mention. Trade groups exist for practically every health care facility safety topic imaginable. In addition, many states or regions have their own health care associations. Health care facilities are urged to make use of the many professional resources available to them through these organizations.

Joint Commission on Accreditation of Healthcare Organizations

With the growth of the voluntary compliance movement, regional and national health care associations appeared across the country. In 1951, several of these groups, including the American Hospital Association and the American Medical Association, founded the Joint Commission on Accreditation of Hospitals (now known as the Joint Commission on Accreditation of Healthcare Organizations). The purpose of the Joint Commission is to standardize practices and improve the quality of care for patients in American health care facilities.

To this end, the Joint Commission operates an accreditation process based on surveys and compliance with standards. These standards, along with general suggestions for rendering high-quality patient care, appear in the Joint Commission's *Accreditation Manual for Hospitals,* which is issued annually. This manual has many helpful suggestions for what should be included in an overall safety program, such as accident prevention techniques, safety committee requirements, and fire safety. In developing many of its inspection criteria, the Joint Commission incorporates the standards of agencies such as the EPA and OSHA and organizations such as NFPA. Compliance with these federal rules provides the foundation for Joint Commission accreditation.

Any health care facility can apply to the Joint Commission for accreditation once certain preliminary requirements have been met. After the facility has paid the appropriate fees and completed the extensive preparatory materials, a Joint Commission team will conduct a survey for accreditation.

The entire accreditation process can be very beneficial, although it is somewhat time-consuming and relatively expensive. The value it holds will have to be assessed by each facility. Should the facility decide to proceed, it will have behind it the full consulting resources of the Joint Commission, a respected, not-for-profit group recognized as a source of excellence by many federal, state, and local governments and their safety-related departments. Additionally, through the accreditation process, health care personnel will learn effective means of limiting risks, lowering financial losses, and improving patient care.

Another approach is to use the Joint Commission's accreditation manual guidelines in the facility and make them part of the comprehensive safety program. Using the manual, the facility can rely on the technical knowledge and expertise of this highly regarded organization, if accreditation is currently not feasible.

National Fire Protection Association

The National Fire Protection Association (NFPA) is an independent, not-for-profit organization that develops consensus standards for essential fire safety in all building types in the country, including health care facilities. The NFPA draws on expert advice from various fields in developing its codes; it is widely recognized as a reliable source of fire protection guidance. Consequently, NFPA codes have been accepted by the federal and most state and local governments as the basis for their fire prevention codes. The Joint Commission also exchanges information with the NFPA through active participation on NFPA committees.

The two most important standards for health care facilities are NFPA 99, Standard for Health Care Facilities, and NFPA 101, Life Safety Code. NFPA 99 establish criteria for safeguarding patients and health care personnel from fire, explosion, electrical hazards, and related hazards associated with locations where anesthesia is administered. (NFPA 99 is part of over 50 publications that apply to health care facilities.) The sections of NFPA 99 that more specifically apply to health care facilities are Respiratory Therapy, Essential Electrical Systems for Health Care Facilities, Safe Use of Electricity in Patient Areas of Hospitals, Health Care Emergency Preparedness, Laboratories in Health Related Institutions, Medical–Surgical Vacuum Systems in Hospitals, and Use of Inhalation Anesthetics (Flammable & Nonflammable).

The codes for life safety are established in NFPA 101, which considers a number of elements such as early warning detection and alarm systems, fire partitions, exit identification and lighting, sprinkler systems, building care maintenance, and storage for all occupied buildings. Included in the code are requirements for emergency preparedness plans and drills, exit arrangements, portable fire extinguishers, and waste-handling systems. The disaster preparedness section provides information necessary for the preparation and implementation of a facility's individual plan. [*Note:* In some areas of the South and Midwest, the Uniform Fire Code (UFC) sometimes supersedes NFPA codes. Those not sure of the status of codes in their region should check with their local and state regulatory agencies.]

A source of overall information on the latest developments in fire protection systems, equipment, and techniques is the latest edition of the NFPA *Fire Protection Handbook.* An NFPA training film entitled *Fire Safety in Health Care Facilities* also provides an overview of fire protection methods for health care. Another NFPA film, *Evacuation of Medical Facilities,* focuses on successful evacuations from a health care facility.

The NFPA is also a source of training materials of all sorts, including books, pamphlets, posters, slide programs, films, and training manuals for both in-house and home fire protection training. A number of seminars are offered each year, and technical advice is available. An individual membership is beneficial for the person most responsible for the fire safety function in each facility.

American National Standards Institute

In 1918, several professional organizations and government agencies formed the American National Standards Institute (ANSI) to coordinate the issuance of standards by organizations with similar responsibilities. The ANSI's goal is to minimize duplication and conflict among the numerous regulations affecting business and industry. The organization works to assist voluntary organizations and governmental agencies in developing regulations, while also seeking a consensus on the need for standards.

The ANSI conducts a review process by which a regulation or requirement is approved as an American National Standard. In order to achieve this approval, the agency issuing the standard must be able to provide evidence that all those affected by the standard were allowed either to participate in or comment on the development of the regulation. With this approval, the standard is then generally recognized and accepted for use.

Approval from the American National Standards Institute extends to regulations affecting health care as well. In addition, through its approval process ANSI ensures that when the health care industry is affected by a regulation, it has a say in the standard's development. Health care managers and administrators should make use of this opportunity to contribute to the process by which standards that directly affect them are developed.

Compressed Gas Association

Health care facilities routinely use a number of compressed gases throughout the facility, including ethylene oxide, anesthetic gases, and oxygen. Because these gases are stored under tremendous pressure, even minimal disturbance can cause this pressure to be released in a destructive manner. If not handled and stored with great caution, compressed gases pose a very serious danger of explosion, injury, and property damage.

The Compressed Gas Association (CGA) was founded in 1913 as a not-for-profit trade association representing the compressed gas industries. It provides technical advice and safety coordination for businesses in these industries. However, the CGA is also concerned with the handling of compressed gases wherever they are used, including in health care facilities. It provides a variety of services to users of compressed gases, including technical publications and audiovisual materials. The CGA also advises the NFPA in developing compressed gas standards. The CGA is an excellent source of information on the safe use of compressed gases.

☐ Comparing Applicable Regulations

As this chapter has shown, the voluntary standards and governmental regulations affecting health care are many and various. Table 6-3 summarizes the agencies and voluntary organizations discussed herein and their scope. Moreover, requirements are often duplicated by several agencies. Even worse, different agencies may publish rules or guidelines that actually conflict. Compounding the problem is the rapid pace at which some requirements grow and change, particularly those on hazardous/infectious wastes.

The sheer number and complexity of requirements, however, become less threatening if viewed in the right light. Many of the regulations overlap because the responsibilities of the various agencies overlap. For example, both the CDC and the EPA publish guidelines on infectious waste management, and NFPA codes are integrated into Joint Commission accreditation criteria. Understanding these examples will help in learning to view the legislation and guidelines as a manageable body of requirements.

In addition, part of the reason for any discrepancies that exist among the rules is the relative newness of the problems, especially in hazardous and infectious materials regulations. Governmental agencies are learning to work in concert on these concerns as they gain greater experience in dealing with conflicting standards.

☐ Summary

Most compliance organizations work to make information and assistance available to those who need it. Many regulatory officials realize that their standards may seem confusing and try to enhance understanding through publications, training, and direct mailings. These agencies can also be contacted by mail or telephone with questions or concerns, and many agencies operate hotlines on specific topics. Concerned personnel who are willing to take the time will find that using the many resources at their disposal will make regulations less daunting and compliance an achievable goal.

Table 6-3.   Summary of Agencies and Voluntary Organizations and Their Scope

Governmental Agency	Scope
1. Occupational Safety and Health Administration (OSHA)	Workplace safety and health
2. U.S. Environmental Protection Agency (EPA)	Control of the release of harmful materials into the environment
3. Centers for Disease Control (CDC)	Control and prevention of disease
4. U.S. Food and Drug Administration (FDA)	Supervision of the development, testing, and monitoring of food, drugs, and medical devices
5. U.S. Nuclear Regulatory Commission (NRC)	The handling, use, and disposal of radiological materials
6. State and local agencies	Worker's compensation (many areas also covered by federal agencies)

Voluntary Organization	Scope
1. Joint Commission on Accreditation of Healthcare Organizations (Joint Commission)	Standardization of practices to ensure high-quality patient care; accreditation
2. National Fire Protection Agency (NFPA)	Prevention of fire through standards and technical support
3. American National Standards Institute (ANSI)	Coordination and approval of standards
4. Compressed Gas Association (CGA)	Services to users of compressed gases

Source: *Safety Guide for Health Care Institutions*, 4th ed., published by American Hospital Publishing, Inc., copyright 1989, p. 25.

Chapter 7

Telecommunications

Nancy Aldrich

☐ Overview

Responsibility for telecommunications differs among health care facilities. Large facilities usually have a full-scale telecommunications department to cover voice, data, image, and video communications. Image communications include fax, X-ray transmission, magnetic resonance imaging (MRI), and so forth. Video communications include video conferencing, security monitors, live satellite educational broadcasts, patient entertainment networks, and so forth. Typically, the telecommunications department also is responsible for the hardware, the software, and the lines to provide communications services.

In most facilities, however, several departments are responsible for telecommunications. Principal responsibility may fall into a seemingly unrelated area. The main departments with full or partial responsibility for telecommunications include plant engineering, facilities management, administrative services, and information systems. Other departments that may have partial responsibility for telecommunications include auxiliary services, security, clinical engineering and finance/accounting.

The placement of telecommunications responsibilities within a health care facility depends on the size of the facility, the number and size of the facility's remote locations, the extent of the geographical area supported by the facility, and the facility's involvement in activities. These activities may require remote access, such as community education, physician referral services, and shared-information systems.

For the purpose of addressing telecommunications within a health care facility, the following information assumes that the responsibility for telecommunications rests primarily within a single department.

☐ Department Head Responsibilities

Typically, a director or manager heads the telecommunications responsibilities within a health care facility. In large facilities, several managers may be individually responsible

The author wishes to acknowledge the assistance of James H. Geiss, M.A., in the preparation of this chapter. Mr. Geiss is a senior consultant with Computer Task Group's Telecommunications Management Consultants, Needham, Massachusetts.

for various telecommunications functions, such as voice communications, data communications, or networks.

Ideally, the telecommunications director should develop a charter that defines the scope of the telecommunications department's responsibilities and performance expectations. The primary responsibilities of the director are to:

1. *Manage daily staff efforts:* Staff may include operators, coordinators, trainers, technicians, and analysts. The director also coordinates the interaction of telecommunications personnel with the staff and management of other departments.
2. *Establish and manage cost control measures:* The director provides periodic cost reporting to immediate and upper management, and monitors bills from carriers, telephone utilities, and vendors. If requested, he or she provides costs on charge-backs to departments that incur telecommunications expenses.
3. *Set performance standards for telecommunications systems and networks:* These standards may include system uptime, speed of answering, frequency of busy signals, and other yardsticks.
4. *Monitor performance of systems and networks:* The telecommunications director negotiates appropriate remedial and preventive maintenance contracts with external vendors and monitors the performance of vendors in fulfilling the contract. Occasionally, the director manages the technical staff who perform maintenance.
5. *Manage the installation and rearrangement of telephone and data communications connections for other departments:* Telecommunications assists other departments in defining reasonable expectations for service. After explaining the capabilities of the facility's networks, systems, and instruments, the telecommunications director provides assistance in designing and revising other departments' communications setups.
6. *Develop and revise departmental disaster plan:* The plan should include prevention, preparedness, recovery, and alternative fallback for mission-critical systems and key users.
7. *Oversee the monitoring of security equipment:* Switchboard operators may have responsibility for monitoring video screens and alarms and alerting security of any problems.
8. *Develop an annual capital and expense budget:* The budget shows the total capital value of all telecommunications hardware and total expenditures on lines, calls, service, staff, and other entries.
9. *Manage the installation of new systems:* The director manages the process by which the department designs, specifies, selects, and implements new telecommunications systems and networks that provide internal and external communications.
10. *Be part of the facility's management team:* The telecommunications director needs to be aware of the facility's strategic plan. Performance of telecommunications responsibilities should reflect the hospital's overall goals and objectives.
11. *Participate in the design, specification, selection, and implementation of related systems that interface with or affect the facility's telecommunications systems and networks:* For example, the telecommunications director may be part of a task force to select a new information system or security alarm system.

☐ Staffing

Within a health care facility, personnel reporting to the telecommunications department may include switchboard operators, coordinators, technicians, telecommunications analysts, trainers, and clerical staff. Outside vendors may be used for some tasks.

- *Switchboard operators:* Often the duties of switchboard operators on one or more shifts are combined with those of a receptionist. The position may also utilize reception personnel as a backup resource. Even facilities with automated attendant services require at least one operator for callers who need assistance with extensions or callers without touch-tone telephones.

The primary responsibilities of switchboard operators or attendants are to receive and distribute incoming calls and to properly route inquiries by physicians, insurers, suppliers, families of patients, members of the community, and others. Secondary duties may include updating directories or keeping logs. In some facilities, operators also monitor security alarms and video screens.

- *Coordinators of large networks and systems:* Most telephone systems, also known as private branch exchanges (PBXs), require at least one part-time system administrator or coordinator. (The terms *system administrator* and *network administrator* will be used throughout this chapter to refer to the position that is responsible for the day-to-day administration of a major network or system. This is the common title in telecommunications circles and should not be confused with the traditional administrator or assistant administrator position in a hospital.) The system coordinator performs software updates and changes, develops and analyzes traffic reports, processes user requests, handles vendors' work orders, manages expense charge-backs, updates directories, and keeps records. A hospitalwide backbone data network or an external network supporting remote sites or physicians may also demand a full- or part-time network administrator or coordinator. System administration can include paging, voice mail, and physicians' answering systems.

- *Technicians:* A telecommunications department can include technicians who provide maintenance and installation services for the communications systems and networks. Often a mid-sized system or network can economically justify the support of full-time technicians or the training of electronic technicians from other departments. Technicians from such departments as facilities management, clinical engineering, and biomedical engineering frequently support telephone and data systems.

For several reasons, internal technicians are used more for installations and moves than for pure maintenance. Because installations and moves can be easily scheduled as a flat work load (during slow times), they are not as demanding as maintenance. During installations and moves, on-the-job training is easier, and the telecommunications department can save the expense of outside vendor charges.

- *Telecommunications analysts:* Telecommunications analysts, usually used only by large hospitals and health care chains, have several functions. They perform large system selection and upgrade studies, analyze telecommunications industry trends related to health care, appraise the financial value and employee productivity of existing systems, and provide technological input to information systems projects. The telecommunications manager or an experienced system administrator can also perform the duties of the telecommunications analyst.

- *Trainers:* Trainers are used in large facilities that have many new users on systems and networks. Trainers are also utilized when members of the external community, such as physicians and clinical staff, use the facility's network.

Trainers are responsible for conducting training sessions for end users on the proper use of features on any of the following: telephone system, voice mail, paging, physician registry, local area network, remote data access network, and so forth. They also perform one-on-one training for new employees and physicians, refresher training classes for all users, and advanced training for more sophisticated users. Methods of instruction include individual, classroom, or small department groups.

- *Clerical support:* A large telecommunications department may have its own clerical staff. This staff supports all functions and groups by keeping traffic records and statistics, assisting with billing reviews, providing data entry to administrative data bases, and keeping drawings up to date. Duties also include routine clerical functions such as typing, filing, and answering telephones. Often they are the answering point for receiving work orders and trouble reports.

☐ Considerations in Determining Staffing

Key issues in determining staffing requirements, staff selection, and staff management include:

- *Cross-training:* Because the telecommunications department is usually small, personnel must often have the knowledge and skill to back up other areas within the department. For example, coordinators with knowledge of PBXs and backbone data network administration tools may also back up the switchboard. Many employees perceive cross-training as a positive career benefit, and telecommunications management should encourage career growth for personnel through cross-training.
- *Balancing reductions and increases:* Savings that result from good telecommunications management can be rewarded by additional equipment or personnel. For example, if installation of an automated attendant system reduces off-shift operators, management may approve a part-time coordinator for continued successful performance and effective records management.
- *Backup by other departments:* The telecommunications department should have access to well-trained backup personnel for critical missions, such as high service peaks and challenging conditions.
- *Performance standards:* The telecommunications department needs to establish realistic performance thresholds. For example, operators may be expected to answer 90 percent of all calls within four rings, rather than 100 percent. Alternatively, the uptime objective might be set at 99.5 percent, rather than 100 percent.
- *Multilocation differences:* Requirements for managing a single-building health care facility differ from those for managing an institution with satellite clinics, outpatient centers, medical office buildings, or sister facilities. Adjustments in staffing levels are often justified by the complexity of the network, rather than the size and mission of the facility.

☐ Specific Tasks Done within the Department

Tasks performed by the telecommunications department require a variety of technical, administrative, and managerial skills. Tasks may be performed by telecommunications staff members, other staff under the supervision of telecommunications, external vendors, or a combination of the three. These tasks include the following:

1. Selection of systems, network topologies, hardware components, administrative software, instruments, service suppliers, and long-distance service carriers. (Figure 7-1 shows factors to weigh in selecting large systems.)
2. Detailed analysis of telephone bills, traffic information, system usage, and supplier expenditures.
3. Installation management of large systems and networks. This includes individual components such as cabling, instruments, wall jacks, line cards, or modems. In some facilities, the telecommunications department oversees the work of vendors and other departmental employees; in other cases, the actual installations are performed by telecommunications personnel.
4. Daily management and administration of networks, systems, and information.

Figure 7-1. Factors to Weigh When Considering Bids from Vendors

```
1. Financial Strength
      Bondability of vendor ....................................... 2%
      Financial strength of company ............................ 3%

2. Technology
      Flexibility ................................................. 5%
      Adaptability ............................................... 5%
      Features ................................................... 5%

3. Support
      Project management ........................................ 3%
      Training plan .............................................. 4%
      General continuing support ............................... 10%

4. Experience
      With health facilities of similar size .................... 5%
      Principal/supervisory personnel experience ............... 2%

5. References
      General quality and workmanship .......................... 5%
      System performance ........................................ 3%
      Maintenance ............................................... 5%
      Due date performance ...................................... 2%
      Client/vendor working relationship ....................... 2%

6. Cost
      Bid price ................................................. 15%
      Cost of options ........................................... 5%
      Expansion costs ........................................... 2%
      Continuing costs .......................................... 5%
      Maintenance costs ........................................ 10%
      Unit pricing .............................................. 2%

   Total ................................................... 100%
```

Source: Computer Task Group/Telecommunications Management Corp., 1990. Reprinted, with permission, from *Health Facilities Management*, Vol. 3, No. 11, p. 21, copyright Nov. 1990, American Hospital Publishing, Inc.

5. Service coordination of networks, systems, and components. This includes preventive maintenance; response to trouble reports; diagnosis, repair, and postinstallation acceptance testing; as well as logging and record keeping of services.

6. Evaluation of suppliers, carriers, and service providers.

7. Negotiation of items such as purchase contracts, component prices, delivery schedules, and service contracts.

8. Monitoring of system and network performance.

9. Reporting in summary form to management on costs, performance, problem response, management information, traffic statistics and trends, departmental usage, external usage of services, and other variables.

10. Training of all users and telecommunications staff.

11. Budget planning for the telecommunications department.

12. Budget input to departments who use and are charged for telecommunications services.

13. Answering of incoming calls and inquiries.

14. Monitoring and exception reporting for safety and security alarms and video screens.

15. Resale of telephone services, including long-distance service to patients, visitors, or physicians; basic telephone service to physicians and medical office buildings; and throwaway telephone sets to patients.

☐ Equipment and Technology

The telecommunications department is responsible for a wide variety of equipment necessary for the facility's voice, data, image, and video communications. The equipment includes the following:

- *Telephone system or PBX:* The PBX is a central switching device that handles all voice traffic into, out of, and within the facility. It consists of a central processor (and backups), equipment cabinets and shelves, digital line cards for external trunks and internal extensions, power supplies, and software for call processing and feature functionality. The term *telephone system* generally encompasses the cabling, wall jacks, distribution frames, telephone instruments, and the switch.

  In many hospitals, the PBX is also used as a physician's answering service. Although sponsoring the service can be costly for the hospital in terms of personnel and equipment, many facilities resell the service or use it as an inducement to physicians.

- *Automated attendant:* The automated attendant is an electronic device tied into the PBX that allows an incoming caller to dial a particular extension or "0" for operator. Other menus can be used, such as "Dial 1 for patient information, 2 for billing, or 3 for education." Some facilities use an autoattendant for incoming calls to specific functions, such as physician referral services or public education registration.

- *Call accounting system:* This is a peripheral system of the PBX that measures incoming and outgoing local calling traffic and long-distance usage. The system can measure traffic and usage by total, group, department, and individual telephone for charge-back to departments or patients.

- *Internal data networks:* Health care facilities have extensive information systems for managing financial and clinical data. Some systems are facilitywide; others are departmental. Telecommunications responsibilities for the systems depend on the connection of the networks. Older mainframe computer systems, often connected by direct cable runs, may be the responsibility of facilities management and may not require telecommunications support. The telecommunications department is usually involved in selecting, managing, and maintaining network components such as servers, repeaters, and taps. The backbone network usually responds to distance requirements from central computer devices. Within the network, there may be departmental local area networks (LANs).

  A less common approach to internal networking is the data switch. The central data switch ties together all systems and networks, which allows terminals from different systems and protocols to access each other and exchange data. Some manufacturers' systems also use the voice switch (PBX) to send data.

- *External data networks:* If the facility's information systems are accessed externally (by remote clinics, physicians, medical office buildings, sister facilities, or corporate headquarters), the telecommunications department or management information systems (MIS) function is responsible for a more complex network than if the network were internal only. The MIS department is also commonly referred to as data processing, informations systems, or systems and computer services.

  Dedicated lines of various speeds or dial-up lines can all be part of an external data network. Each line requires a different type of data transmission equipment, such as multiplexors, concentrators, modems, bridges, routers, channel banks, and other hardware.

  External data networks may also carry voice or video traffic. For economy, a high-speed, high-bandwidth line between two buildings may carry all three types of traffic. Facility selection and trade-off comparisons among multiple alternatives are examples of projects that require a telecommunications analyst or the analytical skills of a manager. Although such projects can be complex and time-consuming, they produce generous paybacks in long-term benefits.

- *Network management hardware and software:* As networks grow larger and more complex, hospitals become more dependent on them for many of their operations. To manage large networks, several data terminals and related software are required. Management systems collect and report data on uptime, performance, errors, data speed, overall usage peaks, and usage by departments. Reports may be periodic but can be real-time to allow monitoring and diagnostics. With management systems, networks can avoid unnecessary traffic congestion, underutilization or overutilization of segments, high error rates, poor response to users, and other flaws.

- *Paging systems:* In most facilities, the telecommunications department is responsible for internal and external paging systems. Such systems may include internal ceiling speakers and the system's central control; internal and external beeper systems; mobile radios for facility vehicles and the related antenna systems; and, in some cases, mobile telephones for physicians. Because these systems require electronic repairs, an engineering department with electronics technicians within the health care facility often maintains responsibility or provides support for paging systems.

- *Security systems and alarms:* Usually, a full-scale security department is responsible for a health care facility's security systems and alarms, whereas the telecommunications department provides some repair and monitoring support. Equipment includes alarm panels, television cameras and monitors, and interfaces to the paging systems.

- *Satellite earth stations:* Large satellite dishes may be used to receive or send educational broadcasts, or for a group of facilities to participate in videoconferences.

- *Disaster recovery/backup equipment:* Disaster equipment consists of batteries sufficient for power outages of one to four hours; uninterruptible power supplies (UPS) for 6 to 24 hours; or backup generators powered by a supply of gasoline, diesel fuel, or natural gas. A shared system of back-up equipment often protects telecommunications, information systems, security, air-conditioning units, boilers, and selected clinical gear. Although facilities management is often responsible for selecting, maintaining, and periodically testing the equipment, the telecommunications department may share that responsibility.

☐ Safety and Compliance

A telecommunications department within a health care facility must comply with regulations in several areas, which include the following:

- *Local fire codes:* A telecommunications director or staff member must be familiar with fire safety requirements and technologies.

    Cabling throughout a facility must comply with local fire codes. In many parts of the country, plenum-rated cabling is required in all areas where a conduit is not used. Air circulates freely in an air-plenum ceiling, and harmful toxic gases are not emitted when the ceiling overheats or burns. Often the fire code may demand that health care facilities use plenum-rated cabling, even if the code does not demand the cabling in other types of buildings. Plenum-rated cabling is two to three times more expensive than polyvinyl chloride (PVC) cable. In some states, the fire code specifies Teflon-coated cable, a variety of plenum-rated cable, which offers little functional improvement and is more expensive than plenum-rated cable.

    Local fire codes may also impose requirements and restrictions on telephone switch rooms, which have many of the same features as computer rooms. These special, enclosed rooms are designed to permit a high concentration of cooling to offset the heat generated by computers, PBXs, and peripheral systems. Requirements vary by geographical area. Some areas still require sprinkler systems, even though water can damage computer equipment. Halon, a system that removes oxygen from rooms to kill fires, is required in other areas. A potentially high level of toxicity can result from the use of halon, however, and fire laws may specify other technologies for fire safety.

- *Local and national electrical codes:* Electrical codes specify additional fire safety ground rules, such as requiring fire-retardant cable in building risers. Codes also specify distances between telephone or data cable from electrical cable to prevent interference by electrical or electronic impulses. Some types of cable and digital equipment emit radiation. Electronic equipment, such as modems and bridges, cannot share closet space with electrical cable. Ground rules change frequently and must be reviewed during any major installations.
- *Federal Communications Commission (FCC) regulations:* All systems, networks, dedicated lines, dial-up lines, and trunks must be installed to comply with the regulations of the FCC and state Public Utilities Commissions. These regulations concern the quality and interference level of signals emitted over the public network. Telecommunications departments should record manufacturers' FCC registration numbers on switching equipment and telephones.

Telecommunications systems must be protected in other ways as well. Just as power systems have backups (such as batteries, UPS, and generators), most telephone systems also have built-in backups (called *redundancy*) for continued uptime in case of the failure of key components. Both the primary and backup central processor or power supply should be periodically tested and exercised to ensure satisfactory performance at any time.

External lines and trunks should have lightning protectors, which are fairly inexpensive and can prevent expensive damage and service interruptions. Proper grounding is critical for the main PBX and its peripheral systems, as well as other electronic gear.

Fallback systems are also important. Most PBX systems have power failure transfer so outside trunks can bypass the system and go directly to critical extensions. Some facilities have small PBXs or data switches in "hot backup" states that operate on separate power supplies.

Because outages in the local telephone company's central office could interrupt service on all external lines, a health care facility should price diverse routing that carries some trunks to an alternative central office. Service through two or more carriers is highly desirable because some long-distance carriers have outages over wide geographical areas. During contingency planning, the telecommunications department needs to compare the cost of the potential disaster to the cost of the solution.

□ Program Evaluation

The performance of a telecommunications department can be measured by numerous methods, including the following:

1. Number or lack of complaints by users. In a recent survey in *Business Communications Review,* telecommunications managers from hospitals and other firms ranked the techniques used for identifying/prioritizing end users' needs (table 7-1).
2. Measurements of the percent of uptime of various networks, links, and systems.
3. Average response time to trouble reports and installation requests.
4. User surveys.
5. Decrease in expenses or minimization of an expected increase.
6. Financial performance against budget.
7. Average response time by vendors.

Table 7-1. Techniques for Identifying and Prioritizing End-User Needs

Techniques (in Rank Order by Value)	Percentage of Respondents
Personal meetings with department heads from end-user organizations	89.3% (291)
Personal meetings with groups of end users	86.2% (281)
Monitoring end-user complaints/problems with existing products and services	94.5% (308)
Periodic walk-throughs of end-user organizations to see how things are done	69.3% (226)
Written surveys	52.8% (172)
Review of end-user budgets to see how costs can be managed more effectively	27.9% (91)
Other	10.1% (33)

Source: Reprinted, with permission, from *Business Communications Review,* published by BCR Enterprises, copyright Nov. 1990, p. 41.

Note: The numbers in parentheses indicate total user responses. Percentages total more than 100 because of multiple responses.

8. Mean time between failures (MTBF) on selected components.
9. Grade of service on incoming or outgoing trunks, measured as a percentage of attempts without a busy signal or no dial-tone condition.
10. Number or percentage of calls answered in a specific number of rings; percentage of calls abandoned (hung up before response); percentage of busy signals.

A telecommunications manager may set performance goals, in concert with general goals set by management, in relation to the above conditions. Specifically, a department may be targeted to do the following:

- Reduce costs, contain costs, or hold down increases by a specific percentage.
- Shorten response time to trouble calls, measured by initial response or how quickly they are resolved. Different thresholds may be set for major and minor problems.
- Increased uptime on links and systems.
- Improvement in percentage of calls answered in a specific number of rings, or reduction in the number of abandoned calls or busy signals.
- Increased number of users trained on features or network usage.

A number of techniques can improve targeted areas. For example, vendors can be challenged and tougher service contracts can be negotiated to improve the level of service, response time, and pricing on components. Management or materials management, legal, or purchasing departments can assist in negotiations.

Maintenance quality may be improved in other ways as well. The telecommunications department can schedule more frequent preventive maintenance to reduce the likelihood of major failures. More frequent network testing or better monitoring of network conditions may be appropriate. Because the department may incur increased investments in staff, vendor fees, software for monitoring, or diagnostic equipment, investments should be compared with the cost impact of potential improvements.

Many problems can be abated by better staff training. Without staff personnel trained on telephone system maintenance, for example, an outside vendor must arrive before repairs can begin. Sufficient training to improve diagnostic capabilities is a wise investment, and better cost-monitoring techniques can improve performance against budget.

☐ Summary

The responsibility for telecommunications within a health care facility may be the function of a single telecommunications department or distributed among several departments. The typical telecommunications department is staffed by a telecommunications director whose responsibilities include staff management, cost control measures, and the coordination and design of telecommunications systems.

The staff of a telecommunications department may include switchboard operators, network coordinators, technicians, telecommunications analysts, trainers, and clerical help. In small facilities, the telecommunications staff is often supported by personnel from other departments, such as security personnel, electronic technicians, or outside vendors.

The typical telecommunications department is responsible for operating and maintaining a wide variety of communications equipment, such as telephone systems, paging systems, and internal and external data networks. The staff needs to receive training and instruction in operational methods of equipment as well as governmental restrictions and other regulations for safety and compliance.

☐ Bibliography

Aldrich, N. E. Ten steps for developing a telecommunications RFP. *Health Facilities Management* 3(11):19–22, Nov. 1990.

Gasman, L. *The Telecommunications Manager's (Plain English) Guide to Inside Wiring.* New York City: Management Telecommunications Publishing, 1987.

Geiss, J. H. A charter for success. *Health Progress* 71(9):13–14, 19, Nov. 1990.

Geiss, J. H. In-house maintenance of telecommunications systems. Proceedings of the 24th Annual American Society for Hospital Engineering Conference, American Hospital Association, San Diego, 1987.

Hard, R. CEOs take a new look at the CIO function. *Hospitals* 64(11):64, June 5, 1990.

Holmes, C. N. BCR survey: how communications managers meet end user needs. *Business Communications Review* 20(11):40–43, Nov. 1990.

Leebov, W., and Scott, G. *Health Care Managers in Transition.* San Francisco: Jossey-Bass Publishers, 1990.

Poggio, F. L. The RFP: help or hindrance? *Healthcare Informatics* 7(6):43–44, June 1990.

Stokes, M. C. Upgrading hospital phones improves patient service. *Federation of American Health Systems Review,* Nov.–Dec. 1989.

Thobe, D. J. Telecom compensation issues for 1990. *Business Communications Review* 20(1):33–38, Jan. 1990.

Chapter 8
Materials Management

Patrick E. Carroll, Clarence W. Daly, and Jamie C. Kowalski

☐ Overview

The term *materials management* can be defined as the management principles and systems applied to control the flow of supplies and equipment from the point of identification of need for acquisition to the point of disposition. Reduced to basic terms, it is "having the right thing at the right place at the right time at the right price (lowest total cost)." Materials management is a discipline, a body of interrelated concepts and principles similar to finance, marketing or human relations. Although primary responsibility for materials management may rest with a designated individual or within a materials management department, materials management is most effectively applied when understood, accepted, and practiced in a systematic fashion throughout the organization.

Materials management has a major impact on the hospital, both operationally (figure 8-1) and financially. Studies have consistently shown that ordering, procuring, storing, moving, and using supplies consume up to 45 percent of a hospital's operating budget (AMSCO, 1977, p. 27). This includes the time that clinical and support staff are involved in supply systems. The expenditures for the supplies alone are 13 to 23 percent of a hospital's budget, according to many studies and data published by the American Hospital Association. The scope of materials management can be diverse and defined in many ways. A model that organizes materials management activities can be described according to the following types of activities:

- *Acquisition:* Product and source identification, evaluation and selection, procurement, vendor negotiations (regarding terms, lease, and rental arrangement), shipping and receiving arrangements, and equipment acquisition
- *Warehousing:* Receipt and storage of goods, supplies, equipment, and furniture

Portions of this chapter were adapted from Goldberg, A. J., and Buttaro, R. A. *Hospital Departmental Profiles.* 3rd ed. (Chicago: American Hospital Publishing, 1990) and from Kowalski, J. C. *Materials Management: Policy and Procedure Manual.* 2nd ed. (originally published in 1989 by the Catholic Health Association; copyright transferred to J. Kowalski in 1990 and now published by American Hospital Publishing, Inc.).

The authors wish to acknowledge the assistance of Steven Rousso, M.P.A., M.B.A., in the preparation of this chapter. Mr. Rousso is the director of operations consulting at Starcare International in Walnut Creek, California.

Figure 8-1. Model of Materials Management Functions/Concepts

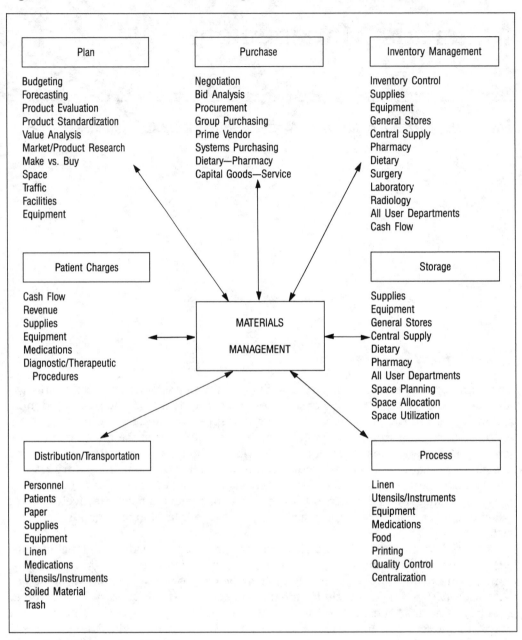

Source: Kowalski-Dickow Associates, Inc.

- *Inventory management:* Maintaining appropriate levels on hand in storage and user department locations
- *Distribution and transportation:* Materials handling; delivery and receipt of product, equipment, waste, messenger and mail service; and patient escort and transportation system
- *Processing:* Cleaning, assembling, wrapping, and sterilizing instruments; cleaning laundry; and producing printed forms and documents

This chapter concentrates on three of the main tasks of a materials management department: purchasing, stores and distribution, and central service. In some facilities, functions such as linen service, housekeeping, print shop, mailroom, patient transportation, waste handling, copier service, record storage, and fixed-asset management are under the purview of the materials management department; however, these are not covered in this chapter. (Linen is discussed in chapter 9, and housekeeping tasks are discussed in chapter 3.) Before turning to the specific tasks, however, background on materials management and information on department head responsibilities, the organizational structure of a materials management department, and staffing will be covered.

☐ The Emergence of Materials Management

Materials management in the health care industry began its evolution in the late 1960s and early 1970s as a direct result of the innovative facility design work of Gordon Friesen, who advocated the centralization of storage and reprocessing in order to make facilities more efficient. His "form follows function" philosophy further led hospitals to evaluate and implement centralization of and specialization in supplies/materials management. In the mid-1970s, Dean Ammer's research profiled the current state of materials management in hospitals; and in the late 1970s, Charles Housley defined a working model based primarily on a hospital he worked for. However, given health care's inclination toward decentralization and the absence of economic incentives for cost-efficiency until the early 1980s, the evolution and acceptance of a centralized materials management model were slow.

The Tax Equity and Fiscal Responsibility Act of 1982 (P.L. 97-248) and the Social Security Amendments of 1983 (P.L. 98-21), which enacted a prospective payment system, provided significant impetus to the acceptance of health care materials management by providing financial incentives for cost-effective operations. Additional impetus was provided in 1983, when the American Society for Hospital Materials Management, in collaboration with Brother Ned Gerber of Coopers & Lybrand, developed *National Performance Indicators for Hospital Materials Management* as the first of three comparisons of practices among U.S. hospitals.

In conjunction with Ernst & Whinney (now Ernst & Young), the Health Industry Distributors Association developed *From Producer to Patient* (1988), a six-month industry research project addressing the distribution of medical products from manufacturer to consumer. The project was conducted to identify labor and inventory redundancies within the supply system. By the close of the decade, materials management had emerged as a profession dedicated to deal with the challenges of the difficult economic environment confronting the health care industry.

☐ Department Head Responsibilities

The department head, usually called the director of materials management, reports to the senior management of the facility and is responsible for developing, implementing, and administering a coordinated supply support system that operates efficiently and meets the needs of the institution's departments and consumers. Specifically, this calls for:

- Developing a strategy for hospitalwide materials management and the structure for achieving its goals and objectives
- Developing policy and procedures in purchasing, inventory control, receiving and storage, distribution, print shop, mail service, materials processing, linen service, and other areas
- Using personnel, space, equipment, capital, and time to meet objectives
- Providing administrative support to senior management in the form of reports, budgets, supply utilization analyses, forms management, and capital expenditure management

- Developing departmental staff through ongoing coaching, in-service education, on-the-job training, and evaluation
- Maintaining good working relationships with all departments by providing service, management assistance, and open communication
- Maintaining adequate operating supply levels in the health care facility and coordinating timely supply distribution
- Maintaining a high degree of managerial competence through continuing education or participation in seminars, conventions, and institutes, as well as field trips to other institutions

☐ Department Head Qualifications

Titles and backgrounds of the individuals serving as directors of materials management are diverse; their previous experience may include work with medical suppliers or in clinical areas, purchasing, or industry. Recently, there has been some growth in the number of individuals entering the field with health care administration and pharmacy backgrounds as well as experience in for-profit industries. An important trait of the director is the ability to develop a systems perspective to envision the total costs in lieu of only product purchase prices.

Sophisticated materials management systems will require strong skills in logistics, financial analysis, and planning. Responsibilities for customer contact and patient satisfaction require solid marketing and human relations skills as well. Although bachelor of science degrees had become the acceptable norm from the 1960s through the 1980s, the complex challenges of today and the future are commanding advanced education and degrees. For materials managers who are talented and prepared, the rewards will be commensurate with the significant challenge.

☐ Organizational Structure

The director of materials management can have a wide range of related responsibilities, and the scope of these responsibilities will help determine the organizational structure of the department. The focus of this chapter is on the materials management organizational structure in which the director of materials management assumes responsibility for purchasing, stores and distribution, and central service (figure 8-2). However, other organizational structures are possible; in some facilities, these functions may or may not report to the materials manager. (In the past, central service was part of the nursing department but today, in most health care facilities, it reports to a materials manager.)

Figure 8-2. One Example of a Functional Materials Management Organization

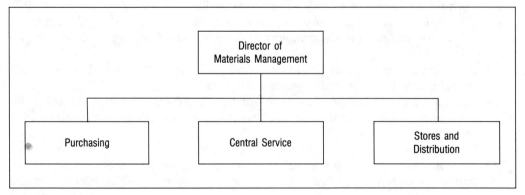

Source: McFaul & Lyons, Inc.

The responsibilities of materials management are basically similar regardless of departmental organization. They are as follows:

- *Purchasing* is responsible for processing purchase requests, identifying product sources, negotiating prices, and conducting product research activities. Its objective is to obtain goods and services, on time, for the lowest total cost.
- *Stores and distribution* is responsible for receiving products, storing, distributing to departments, and delivering goods to their point of use, on time, as efficiently as possible.
- *Central service* is responsible for the reprocessing of patient care reusables and equipment and, in some hospitals, management of the patient care supply inventory and patient charge initiation and reconciliation.

Centralized versus Decentralized Materials Management

Although many health care facilities may organize their structure to provide for centralized materials management, actual practice may be decentralized. In many health care settings, absolute centralization or decentralization is very rare. It is, however, the degree of centralization of purchasing, distribution, receiving, inventory control, and processing a facility employs that determines the level of service and, frequently, the degree of cost-effectiveness that materials management can provide for the organization. Such centralization also facilitates charge analysis and cost accounting.

The centralization of hospitalwide materials functions can yield cost savings as well as facilitate more efficient and effective service. Centralization can enable hospitals to consolidate and control services as follows:

- *Purchasing:* Centralized purchasing can eliminate uncontrolled purchases from such areas as the laboratory, respiratory therapy, nursing units, and the food service department. A reduction in prices can be realized through improved purchase analysis and group purchasing arrangements. Clinical department managers can focus time and effort on their own operations, service, quality, and productivity.
- *Distribution* (including supplies and medications/IV distribution, messenger services, and escort services): Delivery trips can be combined to reduce duplication of effort and save staff time. Distribution systems can be streamlined.
- *Warehousing:* Centralized warehousing (which includes centralized receiving and inventory control) can result in reduced inventory costs, more effective purchasing and distribution, and improved use of space.
- *Processing:* Centralized processing includes better use of staff, increased control over tasks such as sterilization and batch numbering, and leads to enhanced quality control. Extensive use of space in surgery can be minimized and patient care staff can be better focused on clinical efforts.
- *Charging:* Quantitative profiles and cost analyses can be used to develop break-even points for determining what products should constitute discrete patient charges and at what appropriate charge. (More details on charging will be covered later in this chapter.)
- *Cost accounting:* As hospitals monitor the expenditure of resources used for patient care, the impact of materials and supplies becomes a major focus. The amount the hospital receives for the care it delivers is fixed under many payer reimbursement formulas, and the hospital must concentrate on the monitoring of resources consumed by the care process. Automation within many hospital materials management systems and patient accounting systems is enabling hospitals to identify the consumption of supply resources by patient. Through this effort, the most effective resource usage is achieved for all patients.

The centralization of materials management offers an opportunity to improve overall service levels and realize economies of scale by eliminating confusing and redundant activities among decentralized departments. From a management standpoint, there is a clear line of accountability established to simplify and enhance the control process. Decentralized materials management may be appropriate in situations such as:

- Hospitals with a management team that is sophisticated enough to know, understand, and apply materials management concepts and methods individually within the various departments.
- Small rural hospitals for which a materials manager cannot be afforded or recruited. In this situation, it is mandatory that all hospital managers know and follow materials management concepts.

☐ Staffing

Typical positions within a materials management department are as follows:

- *Receiving clerk:* Reviews the paperwork for an order, verifies that the items received match the order (quantity, items, and so on), and checks that there is no damage to the order
- *Stores/distribution clerk:* Issues storeroom items and completes the appropriate paperwork to track issues; may deliver stock to a specific department
- *Purchasing agent/buyer:* Coordinates with hospital staff the specifics of the items needed (that is, quantity, type, size, model, delivery date, and so on) and negotiates with vendors for hospital purchases
- *Central processing technician:* Cleans and sterilizes equipment and instruments used in the hospital
- *Transporter:* Transports equipment, patients, and supplies to appropriate locations
- *Supervisor/manager:* Directs and coordinates specific functions within the materials management department (supervisory positions are typically found in such units as central service, stores and distribution, transport, and purchasing)

☐ Specific Tasks Done within the Department

This section describes the major tasks involved in purchasing, stores and distribution, and central service. The actual work performed by each department will vary according to the needs of the facility.

Purchasing

The purchasing cycle consists of distinct interrelated activities: requisitioning, sourcing, evaluating, negotiating, and ordering. Although sourcing and negotiating are usually familiar cost-saving activities, requisitioning and ordering also offer significant opportunities to improve operations and increase productivity.

Requisitioning

Requisitioning involves user departments determining a need for products or services and communicating that need to the purchasing department. Because not all goods and services can be inventoried and distributed in the same way, several requisitioning systems are used. These systems include manual and automated systems and traveling requisitions.

- *Manual system:* Inventory levels in storage locations (storeroom and/or user departments) are regularly checked and products are requested on a written or preprinted form. This process may be done as frequently as usage, storage space availability, vendor lead times, and inventory management objectives require. Multiple items can be included on a single requisition.
- *Traveling requisitions:* The traveling requisition is used to process repeat purchases of items that are used regularly but not stored in the storeroom. These are called nonstock items. The traveling requisition specifies product, primary vendor, substitute vendor, and unit of order account and subaccount. These can aid both department managers and the purchasing department by streamlining the requisition process (figure 8-3).

  In addition to the ease the traveling requisition provides the requesting department, an important advantage is the price and usage history on nonstock products. This facilitates the opportunity to adjust order quantities and estimate annual product usage and demand fluctuation. Because the traveling requisition is product specific (one requisition per product), departments with large numbers of nonstock supplies may believe the use of traveling requisitions is too time-consuming.
- *Automated system:* Automated systems are computer-generated reports, primarily for storeroom (stock) items, that identify items that need to be ordered along with recommended order quantities. Some sophisticated systems have automated the nonstock item requisitioning process for user departments as well.

Figure 8-3. Traveling Requisition

Memorial General Hospital Traveling Requisition								
Product Description: Department: _____ Account/Subaccount: _____								
Vendor 1:	Name:		Cat. No.		Unit:			
Vendor 2:	Name:		Cat. No.		Unit:			
Date	Qty	Unit Price	Date	Qty	Unit Price	Date	Qty	Unit Price

Source: McFaul & Lyons, Inc.

Sourcing

Sourcing involves selecting an appropriate vendor for the desired product or service. For the vast majority of purchases, true sourcing is a periodic activity because primary and secondary vendors are determined by history, preestablished contracts, or prenegotiated purchase agreements through prime-vendor relationships, group purchasing organizations (GPOs), and so forth.

Under certain circumstances, product sourcing becomes an especially important activity. Capital equipment acquisitions, special requests, and some service agreements are examples of these unique circumstances. Sourcing is primarily the responsibility of the purchasing staff, but is most effectively executed when user departments are involved in assisting to determine product specifications.

Evaluating

Before selection decisions are made, it is essential to fully assess how and how well the product meets the user's need. Hospital materials management programs have begun to utilize a concept from other industries called *value engineering* or *value analysis*. This is applied in a three-step process:

1. *Product (or equipment) value analysis* helps the hospital define the functional needs of user departments and how products can help meet the need. It answers the questions: Is this clinical procedure or process essential? Is it done in the most efficient and effective manner? What type of product(s) will best match the procedure and needed clinical outcome? It also defines functional product quality levels and quantity requirements. It helps determine the *lowest total cost* alternative to meeting the need for the product or equipment.
2. *Product evaluation* is a process that helps the hospital select from among various sources and brands of similar products. It may be a comparison of a new product to a current one or several new products designed to meet a new need.
3. *Product standardization* attempts to reduce the purchase and use of multiple products for the same procedure/purpose. Because redundancy adds cost (procurement, inventory holding, space, and so forth), successful standardization facilitates the attainment of the lowest total cost.

All these steps/processes are most effective when they are followed by a multidisciplinary core group, which champions this effort throughout the hospital. The group is best made up of clinicians, physicians, managers, and individuals from the finance department.

Negotiating

Once a product and a source have been established, an agreement for pricing and terms is developed. This is the process of negotiating. As indicated earlier, most facilities have prenegotiated purchase agreements when a variety of terms have been established (for example, unit price, price discounts, freight, payment conditions, technological upgrades). However, in some cases, unit pricing is still negotiated by the hospital.

Negotiation is both an art and a science. It is best executed when led by a procurement professional from the purchasing staff, wherever possible, along with a team representing the user and finance.

Much of the negotiation may actually take place outside the hospital by the GPO, to which the hospital or a multihospital system belongs. Either of these entities attempts to consolidate the volume of all the hospitals represented and leverage that with suppliers in an attempt to reduce product costs, improve service, or other terms.

Ordering

Unlike sourcing and negotiating, ordering is a continuous and routine process involving translating the requisitioning, sourcing, and negotiating process into a purchase contract, such as a purchase order, and communicating the order to the seller of products or services.

The purchase order is a formal document that may be handwritten, typed, or electronically generated. It not only details information regarding the requested product, vendor, and pricing, but also the conditions of purchase, which are usually standardized by the facility. Once generated, the purchase order may be mailed, faxed, telephoned, or communicated electronically. This communication confirms availability, pricing, and terms.

Although the ordering process is the end stage of the purchasing function, it is the beginning of the materials cycle initiating receiving, inventory control, distribution, and payment approval processes. Efficiency in the ordering process is achieved by prudently using a limited number of vendors and consolidating many items on the same purchase order. Computerized systems simplify the ordering process for buyer and seller alike, allowing for faster turnaround and fewer errors, eliminating the need for both parties to complete data entry. Because suppliers also benefit from such systems, they will frequently provide unit-price discounts or other terms to encourage hospitals to order electronically.

Stores and Distribution

Stores and distribution handles receiving tasks, maintains inventory, distributes products, and maintains records to document transactions and the allocation of supply expenditures on arrival into official storeroom inventory or when expensed to user departments. Hospitals maintain stock inventories in a central storeroom to support user department needs that cannot functionally or economically be met by ordering immediately from suppliers. Although storeroom space has traditionally been located in the basement in space undesirable or dysfunctional for other uses, many hospitals recognize that inventory management results and staff productivity are enhanced when adequate space is allocated to supply storage.

Some hospitals have developed off-site warehouses designed with such efficiency in mind. Small, rural hospitals, as well as large tertiary facilities in densely populated cities, are recognizing that storeroom space may have greater value when used for other purposes. This factor is driving the off-site decision or causing hospitals to consider "outsourcing" product ordering, inventory management, and distribution to suppliers. In effect, the supplier takes over the role/tasks the hospital storeroom used to be responsible for.

These value-added services from supply vendors may provide distribution efficiencies in the supply chain (via economies of scale) that may offset the service charges for more frequent delivery. Just-In-Time (JIT) or "Stockless programs" may reduce costs to the hospital and offer the vendor increased market share by funneling more business to the hospital through that distributor. The supplier typically will only extend these additional services in return for more business, because a critical mass is needed to make the services economical and profitable.

Accepting direct-vendor delivery systems agreements should be preceded by a careful financial analysis of all relevant factors including savings/costs for labor, supplies, inventory, charge capture, storage space, and cash flow. Additional considerations should assess the impact of users and potential change management difficulties. Finally, the facility should analyze the additional work load on receiving and accounts payable.

Inventory

Inventory is the buffer between supply and demand. To the degree that demand can be anticipated and supply guaranteed, this inventory buffer can be minimized. In most businesses, inventory is considered and recorded as an asset until used. However, in health care, convention has typically limited *official* inventory status to stores, central service, pharmacy, and dietary.

The remainder of the inventory, which is stored at the point of use and expensed to the department on arrival, is considered *unofficial* inventory. This is subject to nominal attention. Thus, the unofficial inventory, which can range from two to ten times the official inventory (Kowalski, 1987, *Inventory management*) is a hidden asset. It represents dollars invested in user department inventory that cannot be used for other purposes (to pay other bills, salaries, and so forth). To the extent that user departments stockpile inventories, cash flow is restricted and holding costs are increased. These holding costs include the cost of money (interest either paid through borrowing or forgone through not investing in some other asset), space, insurance, and, for some for-profit hospitals, taxes.

Enlightened hospitals are beginning to recognize the importance of recording and managing the inventory throughout the hospital, similar to the practice in the storeroom or pharmacy, because of the potential financial and service benefits realized. Targeted goals and potential results can be dramatic, as displayed in figure 8-4.

Advanced materials management programs will both view and manage total hospital inventories as assets and investigate the appropriate use of all inventory management strategies available to them, including:

- Stocking less inventory in all areas/departments, maintaining only an amount on hand that will accommodate expected and unpredicted demand plus the time it takes supplies to be ordered and received. Instead of keeping several weeks' or months' worth of supply on hand, hospitals should be maintaining only enough supplies to last for days or a couple of weeks at most.
- Consignment programs with vendors that provide the inventory but do not bill for, or expect payment from, the hospital until *after* it is used. This reduces the investment cost.
- Just-In-Time or Stockless programs with vendors that, via a contract, provide the space, inventory, order filling, and delivery service that a hospital storeroom traditionally provides.

Hospitalwide inventory targets must be supported by department- and item-specific goals based on analysis of usage and the application of mathematical formulas designed to determine the best possible on-hand levels, reorder points, and reorder quantities. These formulas must take into consideration the hospital's and departments' unique characteristics: labor costs, space costs, ordering costs, and cost of money.

Figure 8-4.   Inventory Turnover, Memorial General Hospital, 1990

Department	Issues	Inventory	Actual Turns	Actual Days	Goal Turns	Goal Days	Inventory	Savings
Stores	$1,200,000	$225,000	5.3	68.4	12.2	30.0	$ 98,630	$126,370
Central	450,000	75,000	6.0	60.8	12.2	30.0	38,986	38,014
Surgery	750,000	300,000	2.5	146.0	4.1	90.0	184,932	115,068
Cath lab	300,000	150,000	2.0	182.5	4.1	90.0	73,973	76,027
Laboratory	500,000	100,000	5.0	73.0	8.1	45.0	61,644	38,356
	$3,200,000	$850,000	3.8	97.0	7.0	52.0	$458,165	$393,835

Source: McFaul & Lyons, Inc.

Note: Central = central service, Cath lab = cardiac catheterization laboratory.

Distribution

Distribution is the function of delivering materials from point of receipt to point of use. As such, it is closely related to both the purchasing and inventory functions. Distribution, and its associated costs, is often the most decentralized of all the materials management functions.

Although distribution activities can be extremely complex in design and execution, they can be categorized into four types:

1. *Fetch 'n' carry* distribution is the simplest form of distribution and, perhaps, the most labor-intensive. This involves user department staff going to the storeroom or central services and "fetching" products when needed.
2. *Requisition and delivery* is the next form of distribution and is a common method of ordering from stores. Departments complete requisitions or telephone for products that are filled and delivered.
3. The *round* system is a less commonly used form of distribution. In the round system, the materials management department conducts regularly scheduled visits to departments to deliver supplies per some predetermined logic scheme.
4. *Prospective replacement* is the most sophisticated form of distribution. Materials management automatically replenishes preestablished stock levels based on historical demand, in turn based on predetermined frequencies and schedules. This provides the opportunity to better manage labor resources involved in distribution and minimizes the time and effort of user department staff. Examples of such systems include par levels and exchange carts, surgical case cart systems, and unit-dose drug systems.

Although many of the distribution activities are beyond the scope of materials management (such as pharmaceuticals and foodstuffs), advanced departments redesign distribution to minimize labor investment in replenishment and delivery. This includes decreasing the frequency of replenishment, changing replenishment from demand systems (for example, fetch 'n' carry, requisition, and delivery) to prospective systems and adopting direct-vendor delivery systems.

Some distribution systems are supported by mechanized materials-handling systems such as dedicated elevators that move carts only and automatically load and discharge carts without human intervention on arrival at the destined floor. Small items that require quick, random transport are efficiently and safely moved via pneumatic tube systems, just like those used at drive-in windows of banks.

Central Service

Central service is responsible for sterile processing (its primary role) and may also handle patient charges associated with supplies and/or equipment.

Sterile Processing

The sterile processing function is responsible for maintaining an adequate supply of reusable patient care items (such as instruments, utensils, trays, and equipment) through effective and efficient reprocessing methods.

Sterile processing is completed by trained technicians and includes the following tasks:

- *Cleaning:* Items must be disassembled and cleaned. Cleaning removes dried blood, oil, foreign matter, and so forth. At this time, notes are made if devices are damaged or malfunctioning.
- *Decontamination:* This is a process in which contaminated reusable equipment, instruments, and supplies are cleaned further and decontaminated (rendered safe by removal and destruction of pathogens and dangerous bacteria) by means of

manual or mechanical cleaning processes and/or chemical disinfection. Many reusable devices for the care and treatment of patients are not required to be sterile.

- *Assembly and packaging:* Clean items are received from the decontamination area and then assembled and prepared for issue, storage, or further processing. Instruments, utensils, linen packs, and other items are then wrapped so that sterilization can take place while protecting items from contamination until they are used. Technicians responsible for these duties must be trained in the proper identification and handling of medical devices, various preparation techniques, and sterilization processes.

- *Sterilization:* Three methods are available for sterilization of medical and surgical supplies and equipment in health care facilities. These are sterilization by saturated steam under pressure, dry-heat sterilization, and treatment with either liquid or gaseous chemical agents. Many materials can be sterilized (such as rigid and flexible fiberoptic telescopic instruments, equipment, instruments, rubber products, plastic products, and so forth) with ethylene oxide (EO) gas. The effectiveness of the process depends on the type of materials that are used in the design and manufacture of the device and the type of packaging materials that are used to contain the device. However, appropriateness should be thoroughly evaluated before considering the use of EO as the sterilizing agent because of the risk of exposure to the mutagenic and carcinogenic properties of this gas. Adherence to regulations and proper procedures is essential for staff and patient safety.

With the increased importance and expense of biohazardous waste removal, there is renewed interest in reusable products versus disposable products. It will be the responsibility of central service to determine whether the total cost of disposables exceeds the cost of purchasing reusable trays and instruments. The quality of in-house reprocessing will also have to be competitive with disposables in order to persuade users to support the use of reusables.

Patient Supply and Equipment Charges

Historically, central service played an important role in the establishment and management of discrete patient charges for supplies and equipment. For patient care supplies, central service and finance confer to determine which products constitute separate charges. Operationally, in either case, central service reconciles charges to usage (therefore, replenishment) to ensure proper charge capture.

With the onset of prenegotiated managed care contracts (fixed payment for hospitalization regardless of resources used), the relative frequency of the full-charge–paying patient has been significantly reduced, causing health care facilities to question the efficacy of processing individual charges for supplies and equipment. Indeed, Medicare and legislation in certain states (New Jersey, Maryland, and others) have virtually eliminated charge-paying (fee-for-service) patients. However, processing patient charges may be prudent for some facilities depending on payer mix.

Some facilities have restructured supply and equipment charges to apply differences in procedural payer mixes to improve net income (Carroll and Gross, 1987). Other hospitals continue processing individual supply charges because it is the only means to track actual usage in detail, thus helping hospitals define the costs of services. However, with the evolution of hospital cost accounting systems and the potential evolution to an all-payer system (all fixed-payment contracts; no charge payers) it is likely that individual patient supply charges will be discontinued. In the interim, however, the decision whether to continue to unbundle patient charges should be carefully considered with the involvement of the finance department (Carroll, 1991).

With the ever-limiting labor resources available to provide services, materials managers must critically assess benefit versus effort expended in reconciliation activities. Reconciliation of patient charges, as with other materials management activities, has an opportunity cost element. Labor allocated to reconcile charges cannot be deployed toward other efforts. To the degree labor involved in reconciling charges can be redeployed to areas where even greater benefits can be realized, the materials manager should discontinue reconciliation in favor of the activity that would realize the greater benefit. Obviously, in an ideal situation, the materials manager would be granted resources to realize the benefits from both activities as long as the benefits exceed the costs.

The Reimbursement Environment

Before discussing whether reconciliation of patient charges is worthwhile, it is helpful to understand some background on how patient charges are made. It would be difficult to imagine a less efficient system to charge for a product (that is, health care) than by discrete itemized detail of every raw ingredient. Obviously, most U.S. industries sell by product (automobiles, furniture, clothing, and so forth) in lieu of units (à la carte). To be sure, business conducts product line accounting analyses to determine costs involved (labor, materials, overhead) and desired profit before pricing their products. However, pricing determinations are global (by product), and unit cost or price is, for the most part, not visible to the consumer.

Although health care is moving toward product line sales (that is, episodes of illness) and, thus, product line accounting, a large part of health care "sales" are still packaged as units (for example, daily room charge, laboratory test, central service product). Thus, to the degree the third parties insist upon detail on bills and, therefore, have an impact on reimbursement, selling health care service by unit will prevail.

The Patient Supply Charge System

The typical patient supply charge system involves identifying discrete patient chargeable products, establishing a price (usually through a markup formula), developing a method (sticker, ticket) to communicate to the patient care provider that the product is chargeable, and generating a charge through the patient billing system. If reconciliation activities are involved, usage is compared with actual charge generation to note variances and make necessary corrections.

This complex system, again necessitated by the reimbursement environment, requires considerable labor intensity (affixing charge labels, removing labels to document patient usage, inputting patient charges, and reconciliation) involving several departments (central service, nursing, and possibly, data processing). Importantly, the charge documentation process is dependent on the individual patient care provider, whose motivation toward patient charge generation may be limited. Finally, depending on the method of charge generation (that is, patient billing summary versus kardexes), interface of the supply issue and patient billing information systems, and perceived and/or actual accuracy of the supply replenishment systems, the confidence in the reconciliation process may be suspect. It is not surprising that, given these limitations, the reconciliation of patient supply charges is occurring less frequently.

Assessing Financial Returns

Reconciling patient supply charges, like many materials management efforts, needs to be critically evaluated to ascertain cost–benefit. The basic question remains: Does the benefit of additional charge capture offset the cost of the reconciliation?

To address this question, the materials manager should identify factors relevant to this analysis, including gross patient supply revenue, current charge capture ratio (if unavailable, this can be estimated by sampling methodology), potential charge capture ratio (at best an estimate; a reasonable goal may be 95 percent), labor necessary for reconciliation, salaries and benefits, and revenue realization.

Several issues regarding this analysis need to be discussed. First, the additional labor involved should include only resources that could be eliminated should reconciliation be discontinued. In the vast majority of cases, only central service personnel would be involved. Nursing and data processing personnel would not, in most cases, be affected to the point of labor reduction.

Revenue realization is the amount of net revenue after contractual allowances and bad debts. Although this percentage varies both by patient and product, an overall realization should be available from the financial division of the hospital. It is important to note that increases in *net* gross revenues must justify the labor involved in reconciling charges.

When conducting financial analyses, it is important to distinguish between one-time costs/benefits (purchase of software, inventory reductions) and ongoing costs/benefits (labor additions, purchase price reductions). Realizing one-time savings by incurring ongoing costs will always be successful only in the short term. We suggest that materials managers confer with their financial managers to ensure that proper calculations and accounting principles are utilized in their analysis. It is both embarrassing and potentially career-limiting to base major decisions on improperly prepared financial analyses.

For instance, in certain parts of the country (Maryland, New Jersey, and so forth) current third-party reimbursement for all payers is predicated on predetermined rates. Thus, the revenue realization from charge capture would be nil. Because the rationale for reconciling charges implies the results are worth the efforts involved, we suggest materials management confer with financial management to reach an appropriate decision. It has been our experience, however, that for most hospitals in most states (with the notable exceptions of all-payer systems of states such as New Jersey and Maryland), reconciliation of supply and equipment charges is still prudent.

The materials manager should also assess informal factors, including the motivation and historical behavior displayed by nursing regarding charging responsibilities. The best-laid plans may go awry because the director of nursing does not feel that this process warrants attention. The behavior displayed from nursing will inform the materials manager whether cooperative effort will be realized in implementing a charge system.

Other factors to be considered include the capability of competent staff who can conduct the reconciliation, supervisory time to monitor the process, and administrative support. Although these factors do not lend themselves to ready measurement, they are nonetheless very important and need to be carefully assessed in the decision-making process.

Thus, despite the continuing infrequency of charge-paying patients, patient supply charge reconciliation continues to be financially prudent for many institutions. Because of the relatively modest labor investment, and depending upon the net revenue realization, reconciling charges still offers the opportunity to improve the departmental and hospital bottom line. Perhaps more important, structured financial analysis of this and other cost–benefit opportunities will ensure prudent decision making.

☐ Equipment and Technology

Materials management services have historically been provided in a labor-intensive manner and have not taken advantage of some of the technology used for these functions in other industries. The competition for capital funds is formidable because of the dominance of capital budget allocation to high-tech diagnostic and therapeutic equipment. Thus, support services departments must develop compelling arguments for capital allocations. Usually, when carts, computers, automated materials-handling systems, or reprocessing equipment are competing with clinical technology proposals, there is no contest.

Bar code technology has been utilized in charge capturing, asset management, inventory control, and receiving functions since the early 1980s. Bar code labeling for products used throughout the hospital was predicted in 1982 to be fully in place by the mid-1980s. To date, only a small number of all supplies are packaged by the manufacturer with bar codes. This disappointing rate of implementation is the result of many factors, including:

- The cost and technological difficulty of putting bar codes on very small items (such as hypodermic needles)

- The failure of the hospital segment of the health care industry to invest in the scanners and computer systems that can use bar codes for supply management
- The failure of hospitals to demand bar codes from suppliers

Hospitals attempting to use bar code technology for tracking supplies must print and apply their own labels. This is a labor-intensive process and, therefore, discourages some hospitals from pursuing these systems.

It behooves the manager to complete thorough cost–benefit analyses and use sophisticated financial analysis methods (for example, Payback, Net Present Value, Internal Rate of Return) to demonstrate the need for investment in materials management–related technology that maintains or improves services/performance while reducing costs, especially labor costs.

The technology applicable to materials management includes the following:

- Computer systems used to manage purchases, inventory investment, supply consumption, and materials management operations (processing and distribution). The most advanced systems include electronic ordering and paying of invoices, electronic data interchange (EDI), and bar coding to track movement and supply cost allocation.
- Sterile processing equipment that is more automated and/or improves the cleaning and decontaminating reusables. Washer/sterilizers, tunnel washers, sonic cleaners, steam, and EO gas sterilizers are examples of this equipment. With the concerns regarding EO, research is under way to develop other means of sterilizing, thereby minimizing or eliminating use of EO.
- Materials-handling equipment applications include basic forklifts and carts for supply movement, more sophisticated automation such as automated guided vehicles (AGVs) or overhead chain conveyors (monorails) that move carts via computer control, cart lifts for automated vertical transport (with cart inject–eject capabilities), and pneumatic tube systems for small item movement. As the availability of people to staff materials management positions decreases and corresponding labor costs increase, automation alternatives will need to be revisited.

☐ Safety and Compliance

In the materials management department, employees are exposed to a variety of potential hazards, including environmental, chemical, and physical. These include the following:

- In the decontamination area, employees may suffer puncture wounds and cuts or "sticks" from needles, knives, and broken glassware. Procedures for the safe collection and disposal of sharp instruments should be reviewed regularly. Employees should handle returned items as if they contained sharp instruments. This type of situation should be monitored closely by supervisors, and problems should be reported to the sending department and corrected. Any broken glass should be swept up and disposed of immediately and properly.

  Floors in the decontamination area are often wet and slippery and cause falls. Slips, trips, and falls can be reduced by using good housekeeping procedures to prevent spills, worn spots on carpets, or loose tiles on floors. Spills should be cleaned up promptly. Color contrasts on the edges of steps, loading docks, and ramps enable employees to see potential fall hazards. Storage areas should be secured against sliding or collapsing. Step stools and ladders should be used for climbing to reach items stored on high shelves. Products delivered to the decontamination area are often contaminated with bacteria and other microorganisms that can cause illness to the staff. Proper protective clothing and equipment (such as gloves or eye and face protection) must be supplied to, and worn by, employees exposed to these hazards.

- Manual handling of materials is also a source of occupational injury. Sprains, strains, and back injuries frequently occur from lifting, pushing, and pulling. Employees regularly move heavy, bulky, or difficult-to-handle objects (such as large carts, equipment, large linen packs) and should be trained in lifting safely.

  In addition, storage areas should be arranged to facilitate the placing and removing of materials. Principles for reducing lifting hazards should be demonstrated by supervisors and practiced by trainees as supervisors observe them. Training should also include the appropriate use of materials-handling aids such as dollies and carts.

- Burns from steam and overexposure to ethylene oxide (EO) can occur if sterilization equipment is not used properly. Immediate effects from inhalation of EO vapors include respiratory irritation and lung injury, headaches, nausea, and vomiting. Long-term exposure can increase the risk of cancer or mutation in the fetuses of women who are pregnant or of child-bearing age. Health care facilities must comply with OSHA's ethylene oxide standard (29 C.F.R.§ 1910.1047). The standard includes a short-term exposure limit called an *excursion limit*.

- Employees are often exposed to hazards and unsafe conditions in the storeroom. Collisions with falling boxes, carts, or racks of shelving can occur. Safe storage practices include keeping materials neat and orderly; keeping exits and aisles clear; ensuring materials do not obstruct fire alarm boxes, lights, electric switches, fire extinguishers, and so forth; and using bins, racks, and pallets.

Additional safety guidelines include proper attire for specific employees (such as central service personnel). Facility policies will include uniforms or scrub suits, hair coverings, and shoe covers. In decontamination areas, gloves, masks, and eye goggles add to the protection of the staff.

☐ Program Evaluation

Materials managers should not only establish performance indicators to be monitored but performance expectations as well. These are most effectively developed in conjunction with defined user requirements for support, service, response, quality, and so forth.

Departmental Relations

Proactive departmental relations and negotiation of service expectations are important factors in a well-executed materials management program.

Cultivating departmental relations is predicated on a sound foundation and commitment to customer service as the mission of materials management. Involvement in orientation programs (new manager, nursing) provides an excellent forum to discuss materials management's services and procedures. Development of a written statement of services describing hours of operations; names, telephone numbers, and responsibilities of personnel; and departmental procedures further assist user departments. Additionally, regular, informal rounds to departments by senior materials management personnel facilitate problem solving and inspire trust and confidence.

Communication on a proactive basis can further support positive departmental relations. When materials management provides user departments with timely advance notification of order delays, back orders/stockouts, and product substitution, the department can foster understanding by user departments. This interaction demonstrates an attitude of concern for users, whose historical experience with the department may be only during problem episodes.

Materials management departments utilize various methods of determining perceived levels of satisfaction by departmental users. As shown in figure 8-5, surveys provide an

Figure 8-5. Stores Department Service Survey

---

1. Telephone calls to the stores department are handled promptly and courteously:

   a. All of the time _____ b. Most of the time _____

   c. Some of the time _____ d. Never _____

2. The *quality* of items available from the department is:

   a. Excellent _____ b. Good _____

   c. Fair _____ d. Poor _____

3. Products ordered from the stores department are delivered promptly and accurately:

   a. All of the time _____ b. Most of the time _____

   c. Some of the time _____ d. Never _____

4. When a product is stocked out from the stores department, an acceptable substitute is found:

   a. All of the time _____ b. Most of the time _____

   c. Some of the time _____ d. Never _____

5. The frequency of stockouts from the stores department is:

   a. About right _____ b. Somewhat too frequent _____

   c. Much too frequent_____ d. No opinion _____

6. The responsiveness of the stores department to my needs is:

   a. Excellent _____ b. Good _____

   c. Fair _____ d. Poor _____

7. Overall, I would rate the service provided by the department as:

   a. Excellent _____ b. Good _____

   c. Fair _____ d. Poor _____

Major strengths of the department are: _____

_____

_____

Major weaknesses of the department are: _____

_____

_____

Other Comments: _____

_____

_____

Source: McFaul & Lyons, Inc.

opportunity to gauge departmental strengths and weaknesses (Carroll, 1981). From these data, plans for service improvement can be developed and shared with the evaluators. Further, negotiation of service standards may be needed if user expectations are unreasonable (such as one-day lead time for nonstock purchases or two-minute delivery time for STAT orders). Ideally, the survey will be repeated to quantitatively monitor progress and document satisfaction. In addition, the expectations and level of satisfaction of CEOs and CFOs should be solicited, understood, and evaluated by materials managers in order to establish priorities, strategies, and programs that are in sync with the organization and the manager's boss (Kowalski, 1988).

Development of performance standards should be monitored via data collection and audits of both the organization and operations. The criteria or standards should be based on customer needs, CEO/CFO priorities, peer hospital capabilities, and most important, the hospital's own philosophy and objectives.

□ Summary

With the development of materials management as a profession and recognized management discipline, the opportunities available to most hospitals through greater centralization and improved execution and support provided by materials-related functions are being pursued. These include minimized inventories, standardization among users, vendor management, and enhanced purchasing power. Increased computerization and automation now assist materials managers with meeting the hospital's supply needs. More widespread application of materials management concepts is demonstrating the department's ability to achieve the goals of greater efficiency and cost-effectiveness without sacrifices in the quality of patient care.

□ References and Bibliography

Ammer, D. S. *Materials Management and Purchasing.* Homewood, IL: Richard D. Irwin, 1980.

Ammer, D. S. *Hospitals Materials Management: Neglect and Inefficiency Promote High Costs of Care.* Boston: Bureau of Business and Economic Research, 1974.

AMSCO Systems. AMSCO Fact Summary, SC-2533, Mar. 1977. Exhibit 3, p. 2.

Becker, G. E. Formal plan for major equipment purchases saves money. *Healthcare Financial Management* 43(8):26–32, Aug. 1989.

Becker, G. E. Employees, not departments, improve productivity. *Journal of Healthcare Materiel Management* 6(5):42–47, July 1988.

Carroll, P. E. What factors should I consider when evaluating a just-in-time or stockless vendor delivery system? *Hospital Purchasing News,* Dec. 1990.

Carroll, P. E. Six visions of health care's future. *Journal of Healthcare Materiel Management* 7(8):26–28, 30–32, Nov.–Dec. 1989.

Carroll, P. E. National inventory and supply analysis. Proceedings of the 27th annual conference of the American Society for Hospital Materials Management, American Hospital Association, Chicago, Aug. 1989.

Carroll, P. E. Improving materials management with information support. *Computers in Healthcare* (11):64, 66, 68, Nov. 1988.

Carroll, P. E. Inventory control—"cutting the fat." *Pharmacist Entrepreneur,* Aug. 1988.

Carroll, P. E. Creative materials management—doing more with less. *Conference Proceedings,* American Society for Hospital Materials Management, Aug. 1988.

Carroll, P. E. Measuring consumer satisfaction with materials management. *Hospital Purchasing Management,* 6, Nov. 1981.

Carroll, P. E., and Golan, J. M. What to do when the consultant comes. *Hospital Materials Management Quarterly* 11(4):42–48, May 1990.

Carroll, P. E., and Gross, P. Optimizing hospital revenues. *Hospital Materials Management* 12:5, May 1987.

Carroll, P. E. and Kieswetter, B. Comparative supply costs and inventory levels for California hospitals. *Newsbrief,* June 1990.

Carroll, P. E., and Rousso, S. Does reconciling changes still make sense? *Journal of Healthcare Materiel Management,* 1991 (in press).

CFOs say materials managers need more progressive style. *Hospital Materials Management* 14(9):15, Sept. 1989.

Danielson, N. E. *Ethylene Oxide Use in Hospitals: A Manual for Health Care Personnel.* 2nd ed. Chicago: American Hospital Publishing, 1986.

From Producer to Patient. Washington, DC: Health Industries Distributors Association and Ernst & Whinney, 1988.

Housley, C. E. *Hospital Materiel Management*. Germantown, MD: Aspen Systems Corp., 1978.

Kowalski, J. Material managers need to find that "customer service" slant. *Hospital Purchasing News* 10(9):68, Sept. 1986.

Kowalski, J. C. Use performance analysis to meet MM challenges. *Hospital Materials Management* 13(4):16–19, Apr. 1988.

Kowalski, J. C. Materials management crucial to overall efficiency. *Healthcare Financial Management*, pp. 40–41, Jan. 1991.

Kowalski, J. Execs speak up about materials management role. *Hospitals* 63:65–67, July 5, 1989.

Kowalski, J. C. Consignment purchasing: the cure-all for managing inventory? *Journal of Healthcare Materiel Management* May–June 1987, pp. 53–54.

Kowalski, J. C. Just-in-time for hospitals—so what's new? *Hospital Materials Management* 11(11):6–9, Nov. 1986.

Kowalski, J. C. Inventory management has a positive effect on cash flow. *Healthcare Financial Management* 41:105, July 1987.

Kowalski, J. C. *Policy and Procedure Manual*. Chicago: American Hospital Publishing, 1990.

National Performance Indicators for Hospital Materials Management. Chicago: American Society of Hospital Materials Management and Coopers & Lybrand, 1990.

National Performance Indicators for Hospital Materials Management. Chicago: American Society for Hospital Materials Management and Coopers & Lybrand, 1983.

Chapter 9
Laundry

Sidney Pittman

☐ Overview

A health care facility's laundry department is responsible for collecting, processing, and delivering an adequate supply of clean linen. It uses a variety of specialized equipment and techniques to regularly supply clean linen to every department within the facility.

☐ Department Head Responsibilities and Staffing

The laundry department is supervised by a laundry manager who usually reports to the environmental services director, the materials management director, or an assistant administrator. In addition to the laundry manager, the staff can include supervisors, production managers, washmen, attendants, aides, drivers, ironers, folders, and seamstresses.

The laundry manager is responsible for overseeing the day-to-day operations of the department and ensuring that clean linen is distributed throughout the facility in a timely manner. Within the department, he or she sets priorities for linen to be sorted and washed within an assigned time frame. The manager also is responsible for scheduling equipment to be checked and serviced so that it will always operate at peak performance.

It is important that the manager maintain a good working relationship with his or her staff. Making employees feel that they are part of the organization promotes good performance and safe work practices. The manager provides leadership by using employees' skills effectively, enforcing policies and procedures, and providing an environment for teamwork.

The laundry manager assists the director with the department's budgetary needs and works to stay within assigned budget guidelines. As the laundry manager works to accomplish these tasks, he or she contributes to the overall efficiency of the department as well as that of the health care facility.

A growing trend in the laundry industry, as in many other industries, has been to hire outside contractors. The contractors are responsible for cleaning the laundry, and the facility's staff is responsible for collecting, sorting, and distributing it. Linen may be rented or owned by the health care facility. A cost–benefit analysis is the best way to determine whether hiring outside contractors is cost-efficient for a particular facility.

☐ Specific Tasks Done within the Department

The laundry department's tasks can be divided into the following steps:

1. *Collecting:* Soiled laundry is collected from predetermined points throughout the facility. The frequency of pickup and the location of the pickup sites should be determined by department heads and the laundry manager.

    To minimize contamination and the release of potentially harmful bacteria into the environment, soiled linen should be placed in leakproof bags at the location where it is generated. Special care should be taken by personnel to avoid placing nonlaundry items, such as needles or instruments, in the bags. The greatest risk to health care workers of acquiring blood-borne infections is from accidental needle punctures or injuries caused by sharp items that are contaminated with the blood of infected patients.

    Standards do not currently require the use of covers for rolling-type hampers. However, separate containers are required for transporting clean and soiled linens.

2. *Soiled-linen processing:* Once the soiled linen is sorted, stains are removed, a prewash or flushing is done, and the linen is washed and then rinsed.

3. *Clean-linen processing:* The clean linen is processed, which includes drying, ironing, folding, counting, weighing, bundling, and preparing it for distribution throughout the facility.

4. *Storage:* This step involves the maintenance and control of both active and backup inventories.

5. *Distribution:* A facility may use three basic methods for the distribution of linen: par level, requisition, or exchange cart.
    - The par-level method requires that predetermined amounts of linen be stocked at all times, based on patient census.
    - The requisition method requires using units or departments to inventory and secure linen needs for the next 24 hours.
    - The exchange cart method requires that two carts of identical size be maintained for each using unit. One cart is maintained on the using unit and the other in the laundry. These carts are exchanged daily on a predetermined schedule.

        The current trend is to process laundry on a daily basis. Processing laundry based on a seven-day week rather than a five-day week will greatly reduce the inventory of the linen department and thus result in substantial savings for the facility.

☐ Equipment and Technology

Advanced technology has brought about great changes in the laundry department. Gone are the days when personnel had to second-guess correct settings on washers and dryers. Equipment is now computerized and can be programmed to meet the facility's various laundry needs.

Dryers are now equipped with sensor controls that automatically stop the process when the laundry is dry. They also have reverse cycles that tumble the loads in a way that prevents tangling.

Ensuring that the facility has clean laundry is just one job that computers have helped revolutionize in the industry. Computer programs have become powerful management tools as well. Managers can gather and tabulate data that enable them to identify trends and make the best use of equipment, personnel, and resources.

Laundry equipment can be divided into three basic classifications. These are:

- *Washing equipment:* Innovative equipment changes in recent years have had a dramatic impact on washing equipment. Programmable microprocessors began to change the way laundry was done by giving the operator precise and complete control of the equipment. With processors, operators can monitor 12 to 15 washers from one central location and thus monitor the status of the entire washroom from one display screen. These programs also save steps and time because users can quickly and easily classify linen by degree of soiling, thus allowing the load to be washed at the highest standard possible.
- *Drying equipment:* Available on today's market are complete lines of gas-fired, electric, or steam-heated dryers. These dryers are available with a variety of options that include double-manual timers or computerized controls.

  The gas-fired dryer is usually the most economical. It has an improved design that reduces the amount of gas needed to dry a load of laundry. Aluminized steel burners and high-quality insulation also help to make the gas-fired dryer efficient. For many laundries where steam power is already available, steam dryers may be the more economical choice. One boiler can both heat water for washing machines and provide steam for drying equipment and heat. Electric dryers may not be the most economical, but they do have the advantage of being quiet, clean, and convenient to install.
- *Processing equipment:* This type of equipment is used for ironing and/or folding. Because this equipment replaced the need for personnel to manually process the laundry at this stage, the laundry department has seen a great savings in both time and money. A number of mechanical devices are now used in the laundry department, for example, the automatic spreader, the folder, the steam- or oil-heated ironer, automatic stackers, prefolders, large-piece folders for items such as sheets and bedspreads, small-piece folders for items such as patient gowns and pillowcases, and various pneumatic/hydraulic presses. Generally, this equipment can fold or process laundry up to four times faster than individuals can.

In addition to specifying the equipment used in the laundering process and the actual linen, the laundry department establishes what types of bags are to be used to transport soiled linen to the laundering site. Cloth bags are usually adequate. When necessary, personnel may need to wear gloves and a gown or an apron when bagging heavily soiled items.

The use of cloth bags, which can be washed and reused, will usually reduce the cost associated with single-use plastic bags. Also, using plastic bags to collect all soiled linen may place an additional burden on the laundry service. For example, in some states the disposable laundry bag may be classified as infectious waste and would require special disposal practices that might be costly or not readily available.

☐ Safety and Compliance

Safety plays a vital role in ensuring that patients receive clean linen and, at the same time, that employees are not unnecessarily exposed to infectious materials. The laundry department divides safety into three categories: equipment, chemicals, and general safety.

- *Equipment:* With scheduled routine preventive maintenance, many accidents can be avoided. In addition, employees who operate equipment should receive periodic in-service training on correct operating procedures and the importance of proper maintenance.

- *Chemicals:* Equipment operators also need to be aware of the chemicals used in the laundering process. Many of the chemical products used in laundries today contain ingredients that are potentially harmful. Many products, especially caustic alkalies, give off heat when mixed with water. Chlorinated compounds may react violently with acids. Containers should be handled and stored in a safe manner considering temperature, ventilation, and close-by products. Employees should be well trained in emergency measures, including the use of cold running water to neutralize chemical burns. Employee education plays an important role in preventing unnecessary incidents.

  Topics for in-service training include using safety equipment such as safety glasses, gloves, aprons, boots, and emergency showers; avoiding dangerous exposure to bleaches, alkalies, and acids; reading material safety data sheets (MSDSs); and following emergency procedures that pertain to the department.

- *General safety:* Employees should be trained in basic safety measures such as the proper collection of soiled linen, lifting techniques, hand washing, and appropriate clothing to be worn in the department. Visual reminders, such as posters, can also help employees remember safety measures or think before acting unsafely.

As the laundry department works with the other departments to deliver the highest-quality services possible, it is charged by the Joint Commission on Accreditation of Healthcare Organizations (Joint Commission) to assist in the prevention and control of disease. In addition, the department must abide by Occupational Safety and Health Administration (OSHA) regulations and provide safe and healthful working conditions for its employees. Employees must understand what their responsibilities are and follow them. To accomplish this, the department should provide adequate direction, staffing, and facilities to perform all required infection surveillance and prevention functions. These are key factors in complying with standards and regulations.

To achieve its departmental goals, the laundry department performs a variety of tasks. Soiled and contaminated linen is separated from clean and sterile linen, and the separation is accomplished by either facility design or the management of work flow. The clean linen must then be delivered to the user in a way that minimizes contamination from surface contact or airborne deposits. Similarly, the soiled linen must be collected in a way that minimizes the introduction of harmful bacteria or diseases into the environment. When developing policies and procedures for these tasks, the laundry manager should work closely with other departments to ensure that schedules and methods are efficient and productive.

☐ Program Evaluation

Evaluating the effectiveness of a laundry department involves consideration of quality assurance, laundry precautions, infection control, and the isolation and double-bagging of laundry.

Quality Assurance

To provide a means for recognizing and solving problems, a laundry department quality assurance (QA) plan may include the following:

- Use of protective attire and equipment to prevent contamination of both skin and clothing
- Prevalence walks conducted by the infection control department that serve as visual inspections

- Environmental sampling
- Chemical analysis conducted by an outside firm that includes titration reports to check for correct chemical balances in the wash process and ensure clean, safe linen
- Cleaning schedules
- Liaison with the hospital QA committee
- Documentation and follow-up on incident reports
- Patient evaluations and surveys
- Annual inventory of linens

Laundry Precautions

The risk of actual disease transmission from soiled linen has been shown to be very negligible. Hygienic and commonsense storage and handling of soiled linen are good preventive measures.

Soiled linen should be handled as infrequently as possible in order to prevent microbial contamination to the air. All soiled linen should be bagged in the location where it is used. Linen soiled with blood or body fluids should be transported in leakproof bags. Initial orientation and continuing education and training of employees should include epidemiology, modes of transmission, prevention of HIV and other blood-borne infections, and the need for universal blood and body fluids precautions for patients.

Infection Control

Properly engineered formulas and correct mechanical action during the laundry process will result in an almost-complete destruction of pathogenic diseases. For example, hot water (160° F or above) subsequently applied in the final finishing operations further destroys bacteria that may still remain in fabrics after washing.

After the laundering process, the clean linen may become recontaminated with pathogenic organisms through contact with contaminated surfaces or airborne bacteria from employees. To reduce recontamination, some laundry departments choose to treat their clean linen with preventive chemicals.

Isolation and Double-Bagging of Laundry

With the incidence of AIDS and other serious infections on the rise, the need for proper handling of laundry is ever increasing. Many health care facilities are adopting additional guidelines for handling and processing soiled laundry in hopes of reducing the transmission of high-risk diseases.

One such procedure that has developed out of this process is double-bagging. Initially, the soiled linen from a high-risk patient is placed unsorted in an inner bag that often is made of a water-soluble material. When the soiled linen reaches the laundry facility, it is placed directly in the washer to minimize handling. After it is washed, the linen is then sorted and rewashed. This procedure was first recommended in 1981 by the Centers for Disease Control (CDC).

However, in 1985, CDC's research showed that the risk of disease transmission associated with soiled linen was negligible. At that point, the CDC revised its previous recommendations to reflect its findings. In addition, the CDC also felt that by relaxing its position, it was leading the way for facilities to end the practice of double-bagging their laundry, which was an expensive task.

However, double-bagging is still widely practiced. Comparisons made of the bacterial contamination of the outside of the bags of single- and double-bagged isolation linen show the degree of contamination to be similar.

Many laundry managers may justify their practice of double-bagging as being in compliance with OSHA standards. However, OSHA follows the recommendation of the CDC for universal precautions as reflecting an appropriate and widely accepted practice to be followed. These guidelines make double-bagging unnecessary in most cases.

The only time that OSHA recommends the use of a second bag is when contamination of the first bag is likely. With this suggestion, OSHA did not intend double-bagging to apply to the bagging of linen, but rather to the packaging of single-use contaminated items and specimens for disposal.

☐ Summary

The primary function of a laundry department is to regularly supply clean linen products at a given time to every section of the health care facility. This function may be performed in-house or through an outside contractor.

Laundry department equipment has undergone great change in recent years because of a number of technological advances. Two important innovations have been the introduction of programmable microprocessors on washers and automatic sensor controls on dryers. This recent technology allows the laundry department to process large quantities of linen on a continuous-flow basis.

By incorporating technology and promoting departmental efficiency, the laundry department can deliver clean linen to all departments when needed. By doing this, the department not only helps to ensure the highest-quality patient care, but also increases on-the-job employee satisfaction.

☐ Bibliography

Central Finishing Systems of America. *The Centra System.* Charlotte, NC: JRK Modular Finishing Systems, 1989.

Diversey Wyandotte Corporation—International Group. *Servicing Laundries.* Wyandotte, MI: DWC, 1989.

International Fabricare Institute. Laundry operations. *National Association of Institutional Linen Management,* Sept. 1985.

Joint Commission on Accreditation of Healthcare Organizations. *Accreditation Manual for Hospitals.* Oakbrook Terrace, IL: JCAHO, 1991.

Joint Commission on Accreditation of Healthcare Organizations. *Guidelines for Healthcare Linen Services.* Oakbrook Terrace, IL: JCAHO, 1990.

National Association of Institutional Linen Management. *National Association of Institutional Linen Management News,* No. 8611, Nov. 1986.

Norman Dryer Co. *Continuous Automatic Drying—The Norman Way.* Crystal Lake, IL: Norman Dryer Co., 1989.

Otero, R. B., and National Association of Institutional Linen Management Educational Affairs Committee. *AIDS/HIV Guide: All In-Service Program for Laundry and Linen Personnel.* Richmond, KY: NAILM, 1990.

Pugliese, G. Isolating and double-bagging laundry: is it really necessary? *Health Facilities Management* 2(2):16–21, Feb. 1989.

Chapter 10
Food Service

Carol Hart May

☐ Overview

The one constant in today's food service department is change. With increasing emphasis on running the department more efficiently, the focus for the food service manager is fiscal accountability, productivity, and quality.

Nutrition itself has dramatically changed over the past 50 years, including developments such as research findings on diet and cholesterol, diabetes, cancer, and overall health and well-being. Therefore, the dietetic care of the patient has become more vital.

With the advent of Medicare diagnosis-related groups (DRGs) in the early 1980s, nutrition became a more important factor than ever in determining patient care and cost reimbursement. For example, when a patient has a secondary diagnosis of malnutrition, the DRG reimbursement is extended and the patient may stay in the hospital for a longer period of time. Therefore, adequate nutriture of the patient and the quality of the on-staff dietitians become all-important.

Revenue from sources other than third-party payers (patients) is also important. Therefore, health care facilities are putting more emphasis on cafeterias, vending, outside catering, and many other ventures that will generate profits.

☐ Department Head Responsibilities

The responsibilities of the department head, or food service director, are to ensure that nutritional patient care is accurate and timely. Staffing must be sufficient to meet the needs of the facility regarding food preparation and service quality. The director is responsible for overseeing menu planning and the serving of high-quality food (both topics are covered later in this chapter). Other responsibilities include fiscal accountability and human resources management.

Fiscal accountability is one of the director's primary responsibilities. The budgeting and reporting process is crucial as the health care facility plans its overall budget with shrinking third-party-payer dollars. As part of this process, the food service director must consider equipment used in the department and its effect on staffing.

Food service departments rank low on the capital equipment priority list. Usually, medical equipment takes precedence. However, old equipment is often inefficient and costly to maintain. Parts may no longer even be available. In an effort to maintain low labor costs, hospitals will trim personnel in many areas, including food service. This creates a catch-22 situation because the older, inefficient equipment was designed for additional workers, which can no longer be afforded. The food service director needs to be proactive in assessing equipment needs, layout, work flow, and staffing numbers in order to stimulate increased productivity and add new programs, which will enhance revenue.

Because food service workers are among the lowest-paid personnel in the health care facility, they can provide services for patients at a more reasonable cost than the higher-paid professional workers. Such services might include menu selection assistance, early-bird coffee, room service, or passing/collecting trays. By providing these added touches at a low cost, the hospital can be perceived as providing finer care than its competitors.

Human resources management is another responsibility that the food service director cannot overlook. He or she is responsible for hiring, training, retraining, evaluating, praising, disciplining, motivating, and discharging employees.

Often the director finds it difficult to provide a motivating environment for his or her staff. For example, a pot washer who stands over a sink of hot, sudsy water all day and scrubs dried food off pots and pans may believe his or her job is unimportant. However, this is one of the most critical jobs in the department because proper sanitation is essential to the care and feeding of both the patients and the public. The director must make all food service employees aware of the importance of their jobs.

Another aspect of human resources management is providing employee education and training. A well-educated staff will play their part in reducing accidents, improving the quality of their work, and lowering costs associated with redoing work.

☐ Department Head Qualifications

The qualifications of the food service director have a tremendous impact on the food service department. Food preparation and services offered are the director's responsibility. How well the department's services are accomplished is a reflection of the director's basic knowledge, training, and experience.

Candidates for a food service director might include a registered dietitian with strong food management and leadership abilities, a food management graduate, or someone with extensive experience in and financial knowledge of food service purchasing.

The ability to successfully manage employees is another important factor to consider when choosing a food service director. Such training might be acquired through experience, classroom training, or seminars. Past success is a good criterion to use when selecting a director.

The food service director should be energetic, creative, enthusiastic, and able to instill these qualities in the work force. The food service department generally hires entry-level people, with the exception of dietitians and some of the more highly skilled positions such as cooks or supervisors. Workers must feel that their jobs are important. The department head, all levels of supervision, and workers must have a sense of what they are trying to accomplish and how important all their roles are.

☐ Contract Management versus Self-Management

Leadership of food service departments in health care facilities generally takes one of two forms: contract management or self-management.

With contract management, an outside company provides the manager, any assistant managers, and perhaps even dietitians, as well as manuals, educational programs, and financial reporting. The facility pays the outside management a fee for the services it provides (the cost of the provided personnel plus expenses for headquarters and field support as well as the company's profit margin).

The self-managed food service department is frequently led by a dietitian or someone with a degree in hotel/restaurant management and experience in food service in health care institutions. He or she provides management for the department and is on the facility's payroll. About 70 percent to 75 percent of hospital food departments in the United States are self-managed.

The decision regarding which management option to choose usually depends on the availability of a proficient manager and the preference of the hospital administration for self- or contract-managed operations. Having an outside firm provide all or part of the food service management team frees the administration from having to recruit. The firm may provide necessary manuals and educational programs. It should also provide an acceptable quality assurance (QA) program, based on Joint Commission standards. The firm's on-site manager reports to the firm as well as the hospital administration. Reports are generated for the department by both the in-house manager and the outside firm. On the downside, there is often high turnover in the outside firm's management staff as they advance in their careers. Their loyalty is first and foremost to the firm, not the hospital. However, this does not imply an inability to serve the hospital, because their success is measured in part by the hospital administration.

An efficient, effective independent food service director provides continuity, manuals, and so forth, without the management fee imposed by an outside firm.

☐ Staffing

Staffing within the department itself is based on the facility's size, needs, type, and the other responsibilities of the director. Generally reporting to the head of the food service department will be an assistant director for clinical nutrition or a chief dietitian, an assistant director for food service administration, perhaps a catering director, a cafeteria manager, a vending manager, head chef, and a purchaser/buyer. In small facilities, the chief cook, the dietitians, diet clerks (who handle tasks such as menu distribution) and/or technicians, cashiers, and storeroom clerks may report to the director.

The responsibilities of these people vary from one facility to another, but usually a director needs sufficient staff to ensure that the work can be done properly. The span of control needs to be somewhat curtailed so that the individuals supervising the employees can ensure that work is monitored and an environment for success is provided.

Staff under the director include the following:

- The *assistant director for clinical nutrition* is required by state regulations to be a registered dietitian. This individual must be knowledgeable in total parenteral nutrition (TPN) (total nutrition via veins) as well as oral nutriture. A dietitian registered by the American Dietetic Association (ADA) and licensed by the state is required. (However, not all states have licensure.) The ADA provides a code of ethics for dietitians, which serves as a valuable reference for evaluation. Registration of dietitians by the ADA requires that they maintain relevant, current knowledge through continuing education. Seventy-five approved hours over a five-year period is the minimum standard.
- The *assistant director for food service administration* should have a sound fiscal background, know how to contain cost and increase revenue, and provide monthly financial reports to the director. A sound knowledge of food preparation and service costs is essential. This individual must have excellent human resources management skills.

- A *catering director* or *manager* is responsible for generating business, billing, and overseeing service. His or her functions may range from simple luncheons to extravagant catered events for the board, physicians, or the community.
- The *cafeteria manager* enhances the merchandising, provides attractive displays, participates in the pricing of the food, and monitors appropriate serving of the food by the cafeteria workers. To ensure that high-quality food is being served in the cafeteria, this individual should observe at least two meal periods a day.
- The *vending manager* oversees the supply, stocking, and maintenance of the vending machines and is also responsible for counting the funds and making deposits. This position also involves a degree of food production experience such as dating, labeling, and overseeing vending-related business. Food prepared on-site must meet the United States Department of Agriculture (USDA) labeling guidelines.
- The *head chef* is an individual who can prove to be of good public relations value to the hospital. Credibility increases when the chef produces food that is extraordinary—above and beyond that provided by competitors.
- The *purchaser/buyer* is another critical position. This person must comparison-shop to ensure that quality standard for the food are met and the price is the best available for the quality expected. Food specifications are critical in this area, and the food service director, the assistant director for food service administration, and the assistant director for clinical nutrition are responsible for establishing the food specifications. Frequently, larger suppliers have written specifications from which to choose.

The food service director needs to be extremely astute in staffing the department. Overstaffing will result in unnecessary cost to the hospital; understaffing will result in stress and strain on the employees. For example, understaffing may result in work having to be redone because it was done poorly the first time or not done at all. Productivity should be monitored to ensure that the staff is working to its potential.

Clinical patient care accuracy requires that the staff be sufficient to meet the needs of the facility. A general guideline for determining the number of registered dietitians is shown in table 10-1. The mix will vary according to the degree of service offered, the type of services available, the amount of dietetic technician support given, and the nature of the hospital itself. This is only a basis for starting an analysis.

To be competitive with other institutions in their service area, such as fast-food chains, health care facilities are finding it necessary to pay higher salaries even to entry-level food service employees. To add to the problem, there is a decreasing labor pool for these workers. Where hospitals have been adversely affected by decreasing revenues, significant changes in staffing patterns occur—doing more with less and downsizing through layoffs, attrition, or hiring freezes.

Employees are often reluctant to change their work habits. However, lower staffing necessitates cross-training on a wide scale. Smaller facilities usually have cross-training

Table 10-1. Registered Dietitians (RD) per Range and Bed Type

RD	Bed Type	Range of Occupied Beds
1	Medical	50–60
1	Surgical	70–80
1	Nutrition Support	35–45
1	Psychiatry	100–150
1	OB/GYN	100–150
1	Pediatrics	100–150

Source: Reprinted, with permission, from CN Prod Software program, published by Dietary Management Advisory, Inc., copyright 1990.

to a greater extent. Large facilities must follow suit in order to reduce nonproductive time. For example, cashiers may perform a wide variety of functions (such as food preparation, cleaning, or supervision of others) when the cafeteria is closed or business is slack. It is impractical and costly for workers to have large blocks of downtime between assignments.

☐ Specific Tasks Done within the Department

The food service department is responsible for administrative tasks, clinical nutrition tasks, food preparation, food distribution, and inventory.

Administrative Tasks

Administrative tasks that are done within the department include the oversight of food preparation, distribution, and service and other support-related services (such as billing, cost accounting, budgeting, and so on). All aspects of food preparation must be monitored to ensure consistency with what has been ordered.

Another administrative function within the department is billing for services, including any nourishments that are transferred to nursing stations, bulk nourishments for patients, catering services, and services for other meals such as those in the physicians' dining room. The actual billing is usually performed by a clerical staff member.

Clinical Nutrition Tasks

Clinical nutrition tasks include ensuring proper nutriture, helping patients select menus, and providing nutritional education and other dietitian services. Proper nutriture is essential for the on-time release of patients from the hospital. If there is a codiagnosis of malnutrition, plans can be made so that the patient's nutriture receives adequate support and the hospital patient stays in the hospital longer to facilitate recovery. The properly nourished patient will be less likely to be readmitted within the time periods stipulated by Medicare.

Patient menu selection and nutritional education are good tools for helping patients understand what they need to eat in order to stay well and healthy after they are released from the hospital. Patient menus can be used as a teaching tool by describing diabetic diet exchanges, sodium-reduced food, and fiber modifications. When patients are educated, their learning can be reinforced by having them select the menu appropriately. (The next section describes the various options available in menu selection.)

Nutrition education is done by qualified registered dietitians or ADA-certified dietetic technicians. Patient nutrition education can be done in groups or singly depending on the type of diet, the number of times a patient needs to be reviewed, and the patient's general ambulatory status. All the programs within the clinical area need to be part of the department's QA.

One area that has become very popular for revenue enhancement in hospitals is charging a fee for dietitian services ordered by physicians. Many of these services are covered by Medicare and private insurance companies. This adds to the hospital's revenue and helps offset the department's expenses. Such services may include nutrition education conducted by a registered dietitian, calorie counts, nutritional assessments, and many other services that are above the costs generally included in "room and board."

Types of Patient Menus
Patient menus are one facet of food service that need to be planned carefully. There are several types:

1. Patient selection of menu
   a. *Nonselect menu:* The patient has no selection, but is simply sent the foods that are prepared for the day. This greatly simplifies the operation in the kitchen, is less likely to result in food wastage, and will provide the patient with a balanced diet. The pitfalls are that patients may receive food that they do not like and may not eat. Because the primary objective of the food service department is to nourish the patient, eating the food served is critical.
   b. *Partial select menu:* For this menu, only certain patient groups actually select their food. For example, patients on regular diets may select their menu, but patients on restricted diets may not.
   c. *Full-select menu:* Generally, this is the most satisfactory option for the patient. Patients who are eating solid foods, and sometimes patients on liquid diets, receive a menu from which they make their daily selections. A system is needed to tally menus or collect information, so that food wastage is reduced. Only the items needed are prepared in the amounts selected.
2. Menu cycles
   a. *Cycle menu:* Menus usually are cyclic. Cycle menus are carefully planned menus that are rotated for a specified duration, that is, 3 days, 7 days, 21 days, and so forth. The trend has been to reduce the length of the cycle as the length of patient stays has shortened. However, for long-term care facilities, a longer cycle would be necessary to reduce menu boredom. Shorter cycles should result in a highly popular menu and a lower on-hand inventory cost.
   b. *Restaurant-style menu:* One way to reduce food cost is to offer a restaurant-style menu. Food items for this type of menu can be prepared ahead of time and either refrigerated or frozen for later use. The restaurant-style menu is a one-day cycle that lists a number of choices of entrées, side dishes, desserts, and so forth, and remains the same on a day-to-day basis. The modified restaurant-style menu has basic items that remain the same every day, but lists specials that change on a rotating cycle (for example, over a seven-day period).

One consideration regarding menus is the menu paper. It may be as simple as a plain piece of paper with the food items printed on it. Alternatively, in addition to the menu, the menu paper can carry a public relations message including information about the health care facility and perhaps a picture, nutritional data, or other useful information.

Food Preparation

The various types of cooking include scratch, convenience, cook–chill, and cook–freeze. For each type, or system, the relative costs need to be balanced with the overall financial status, mission, and so forth, of the hospital. Convenience goods cost more to buy than ingredients for the same product prepared from scratch. Where labor is scarce or expensive, convenience foods live up to their name. Patient and physician acceptance of the end product is the determining factor in choosing a food preparation method.

- For *scratch-cooking,* raw ingredients are purchased and entrées are prepared from recipes. Most food service departments base their scratch-cooking operation on standardized recipes in order to ensure that the product is of the same high quality for each preparation and so that nutritional analysis for the patient is assured. Because of decreasing labor availability, there is a trend away from scratch preparation.

  Patients and physicians equate *homemade* with *caring,* and this perception must be addressed. Many purchased foods (convenience) are as good as or better than homemade foods because of extensive testing and standardization of product.
- *Convenience-cooking,* or partial convenience mixed with scratch-cooking, or convenience mixed with cook–chill or cook–freeze, is less labor-intensive than scratch-

cooking. Convenience food products such as cake mixes, premade bread, and pans of lasagna significantly reduce the amount of labor required in the kitchen to produce the final product. The initial cost of convenience products is generally higher; but when on-site labor is factored in, it may actually be lower. After all, one does not have to pay benefits to a pan of lasagna. Patient and physician acceptance of convenience foods should be high as long as product quality is high.

- *Cook–chill* is a method of preparation in which the food is cooked in bulk and refrigerated. This method is designed to save food preparation staff labor so that cooks are only required to work five 8-hour days per week. When cooks are working, they are not actually cooking for the meal at hand, but for the next three days. This system requires fewer cooks, but satisfactorily trained workers are needed for meal-to-meal food reheating.

  With cook–chill, food is cooked twice and thus many people object to it as leftovers. If one is using a delivery system where the food is reheated at a remote site, cook–chill is very often a viable option. This system requires advanced menu-planning skills to ensure that foods plated and then heated rethermalize at the same temperature in the same time. This takes time for testing and experimenting.

  A prime advantage of this system is the ability to provide one-shift staffing for most food service employees. Many companies provide a variety of preparation and service options for cook–chill. Demonstrations and tours of existing operations are available. Patient and physician acceptance can vary. Before a complete changeover, however, a trial and extensive education of nursing and medical staffs should be conducted.

- *Cook–freeze* is similar to cook–chill. The primary difference is that with cook–freeze, larger quantities may be prepared and stored in the freezer for longer periods of time. For example, cook–chill food would have to be used within a three- to four-day time period, whereas cook–freeze food could be stored up to six months. Acceptance is similar to cook–chill, but costs may be higher (freezer storage) and there may be loss of product pulled for tempering but not used.

Food Distribution

There are generally two types of delivery systems: centralized and decentralized. In a centralized system, food is prepared and assembled on patient trays in one location, such as the kitchen, then sent on carts or conveyors to the patient areas for service. The trays are distributed from one centralized location to all service sites. Decentralized service may vary in style. Usually, the food is purchased and prepared in one area and then sent to remote locations for service. There might be a commissary on-site with the food sent to several facilities, such as hospitals, nursing homes, extended care facilities, or even schools or day care programs, where it is portioned and served.

Decentralized distribution varies in that final preparation and service occurs away from the preparation site. Distribution from patient floor pantries is common. Here, the food is assembled on trays by a staff member who is trained in patient nutrition and can assemble the tray according to the diet order. Trays are then distributed to the patients on the nursing unit. Another alternative is that the trays are assembled in a centralized location, sent to patient areas, warmed, and distributed by food service workers or nursing assistants. Whether centralized or decentralized delivery is done, any of these preparation methods may be used.

Some facilities specify food distribution as the responsibility of the nursing personnel. This gives nurses the opportunity to prepare patients and accurately record their food intake. On the other hand, distribution by food service employees utilizes lower-paid workers. This method is more likely to get feedback on patient food preference for the dietitians. Also, tray collection is more timely, thus keeping the food service department on schedule. The negative aspect of this type of distribution is that patients may not be ready for the food when it is delivered, and intake information may not be recorded in a satisfactory manner.

Inventory

The inventory process must be maintained on a regular basis, because it is a major factor in determining actual food costs. Internal monitoring can provide information that indicates how well food is being utilized and where wastage or theft may be occurring. Inventory should be taken and costs extended at least monthly.

High-cost items such as coffee, meat, and entrée products should be inventoried more often (perhaps weekly). With a perpetual inventory system, extreme accuracy of daily deliveries and withdrawals of product is mandated. Computerization simplifies this process. Actual physical inventory counts are needed periodically to check and correct the perpetual inventory. The perpetual inventory is the basis for computerized order generation based on parstock levels for each menu.

Overall control of the food purchasing process is key to the success of the food operation. The two major costs in the department are food and labor.

☐ Areas Where Food Is Served

Although patients usually are served their meals on trays in their rooms, some patient areas have central dining rooms where patients can congregate to eat their meals, for example, in nursing homes, rehabilitation units, adult psychiatric units, and pediatric units. Often these patients will enjoy meals and eat better where there are others to chat with and where a change of surroundings makes them feel less institutionalized.

Besides serving food to patients in these areas, the food service department often participates in employee dining programs. A health care facility can offer employees several options: cafeterias, coffee shops, vending machines, or fast-food outlets.

- The employee and/or visitor *cafeteria* should be an attractive, relaxed area that has a pleasant decor, windows, a good view, music, plants, and art. In a very small facility, the patient tray line is used to serve employees after patient tray service. This reduces the staff and equipment needs of the department. In some facilities, the cafeteria is open 24 hours and there is no coffee shop.
- A *coffee shop* that is open the same or different hours as the cafeteria is often used by visitors and employees. Frequently, the coffee shop is open for the midnight shift because the coffee shop can serve the smaller volume with high-quality food at more satisfactory cost levels and in a more cozy setting than a large, empty cafeteria.
- Operating *vending machines* can be done through contracted or self-operated systems. Under a contract operation, the health care facility receives a percentage of the profits. Generally with a self-operated system, a larger revenue is generated. Vending primarily requires a dedicated person to supply and clean the machines. Cooperation is needed from the plant engineering or maintenance staff so that the machines are repaired quickly and downtime is minimized.
- Some institutions have *fast-food outlets* within the building that are operated by a franchise business. The health care facility's nutrition guidelines should be utilized in their menu offerings.

Other service areas for the food service department are physicians' dining rooms, board rooms, administrative dining areas, and so forth. Physicians' dining can be on a paid basis or as a courtesy service. Having a separate physicians' dining room is one way of permitting the physicians to exchange thoughts and concerns about patients without fear of being overheard in the regular cafeteria. It also provides physicians with the opportunity to get away, perhaps to watch television and relax for a few minutes before getting back to their routine.

A fine dining experience in this area goes a long way toward garnering physician support for the hospital. Locating the dining/lounge area near the medical records department may help physicians to remember to sign off their charts. Employees, however, may take offense at special service given physicians, and this must be handled proactively.

Food service catering became highly popular in the 1980s and is expected to continue to remain so in the future. Services provided can range from a simple cart for coffee and cookies to a full-service dinner. Committee meetings, board meetings, medical staff dinners, and other special events may be catered by the food service department. Catering outside the health care facility is often a viable money-maker, but care must be taken that the facility's unrelated business income status is not compromised.

Another aspect of catering that involves patient food service is the room service menu. Room service provided to patients at an extra charge alleviates the institutional aspects of food service. A room service menu may offer deli sandwiches, fresh fruits, beverages, salads, desserts, regional favorites, or hospital specialties.

Generally, this service is available during off-hours, but can also be available 24 hours a day or only when the kitchen is open. It provides patients and visitors the opportunity to get a special meal outside the normal service provided. This helps to reduce the need for ancillary food service operations, such as a coffee shop.

☐ Equipment and Technology

Food preparation equipment includes ranges, ovens, grills, hot tops, fryers, bain-maries, steamers, convection steamers and ovens, and broilers. For a cook–chill operation, the department will need tumblers, chillers, and bulk cookers. Storage area equipment will need to include refrigerators and freezers that are designed for easy accessibility, especially with carts.

Small items such as mixers, food processors, blenders, and slicers are used daily within the department. All these items must be commercial-grade and rated to meet the standards set by the National Sanitation Foundation.

There are many other pieces of minor equipment and utensils, pots and pans, and small pieces of equipment such as serving utensils with plastic or rubberized handles to help prevent burns. Other food service equipment includes tray lines, steam tables, air-curtain refrigerators, salad bar/soup stations, cash registers, and carts.

The tray line itself may be a table in a small kitchen. In larger facilities, there may be a mechanized tray line that moves at a set pace to ensure productivity. A circular tray line uses less space and facilitates tray makeup by its compact design and the positioning of workers. A mechanized line can be stopped and started only by the person checking the accuracy of the trays to ensure that productivity is maintained. Air-curtain refrigerators at the tray line help keep food cold during the service period.

Steam tables for hot food should hold hot water and have built-in drains to ensure safe and sanitary maintenance. In the cafeteria or employee serving area, there is often a salad bar/soup station or deli bar. Facilities may want to consider the possibility of potential infection and cross-contamination before installing one of these units. Anytime customers serve the food themselves, they may contaminate it with the bacteria on their hands. Other individuals may then be infected as a result.

Cash registers range from the simple to the complex. Computerized models are available that hook into the department's computer system and give readouts by meal period, hour, and food served. The computerized registers can be very helpful in controlling costs and comparing the amount prepared with the amount actually sold and left over.

A variety of carts are needed to support food service areas. For durability and sanitation, they are generally made of stainless steel and equipped with large casters that help the carts roll easily on carpeted hallways.

Computerized Equipment

The use of computers is expected to grow over the next few years. Computers now help staff members prepare menus, do paperwork, and maintain production records. Computer hardware and software needs can be determined by the complexity of the operation, the health care facility itself, the on-site programmers, and the expertise of the food service director and support staff.

Nutritional support software that analyzes menus for nutrient content and cost is available. This software can play an important role in helping the department be more cost-effective. Menus can be readily adjusted to ensure appropriate nutrient levels at the best cost.

Purchasing is another area where computers are useful. Computerization can help in tabulating and ensuring that food is purchased as needed. Many departments prefer to use a personal computer that does not have to be tied to the hospital's main computer for daily tasks, such as those done by the purchasing or accounting department. A wide variety of software is available if the facility cannot provide on-site programming.

Robotics have been developed that are capable of doing simple, routine tasks such as food chopping, placing silverware in bags, and other one- and two-movement operations. Although robots that do these tasks may not become popular in health care facilities, they may be used by other support companies to reduce the cost of pre-prepared products that are sold to facilities.

Smart delivery carts that are programmed to travel throughout the health care facility may be another way to reduce labor costs. These carts can be programmed to go to designated areas and return on a specific schedule. Tray delivery carts for cook–chill service are delivered to patient service areas prior to the meal, plugged in, and programmed to start reheating. For example, breakfast may be set up the day before, delivered to the patient area, and programmed to start reheating at 6:00 a.m., to be ready between 6:30 and 7:00 a.m. Breakfast can then be served to the patients when they are ready and the nursing personnel have time.

☐ Safety and Compliance

To ensure that the food service department delivers the best-quality service possible, the director needs to be aware of the various regulatory agencies and organizations that set the guidelines for health care facilities. Many of these are national agencies, such as the Occupational Safety and Health Administration (OSHA); but more specifically, state and local health departments have regulations that the food service department must practice and follow.

These standards include such items as hair restraints, personal hygiene, back-flow devices on the water source, temperature maintenance, cleanliness, and so forth. Food service directors and their staff must be trained and attuned to meet these regulations. The director may request information from these agencies, if needed.

The Joint Commission on Accreditation of Healthcare Organizations (Joint Commission) offers accreditation to facilities. The standards set by the Joint Commission should be an integral part of the facility's day-to-day operations. Many Joint Commission requirements are similar to those of the state and local health departments.

Safety and Sanitation

It is extremely critical that the food service director and the entire staff monitor safety and sanitation. Employee safety must be taught routinely and monitored regularly. All employees must know how to prevent falls, avoid lifting injuries, use knives and sharp instruments safely, and report equipment that is malfunctioning or out of order.

Food service sanitation requires constant care and attention. With so many diseases that are immune-suppressed, and with treatments that affect immunity (such as chemotherapy for cancer patients), food safety is critical. Food must be obtained from sources that are federally inspected and free of disease. Fresh food and vegetables need to be washed carefully in order to ensure that all dirt is removed. In many instances, immune-suppressed patients cannot receive fresh fruits and vegetables because of the potential danger of their receiving harmful bacteria. Refrigeration must hold food at between 30° F and 40° F. Food heated for serving must be 140° F or more to ensure safety.

Sanitation of equipment, floors, and walls needs to be delegated to individuals working in the area or to a porter. Daily cleaning is essential; and special projects for weekly, monthly, and annual cleaning must also be scheduled.

Infection Control

Infection control and education cannot be minimized. It is imperative that the infection control nurse participate in training so that employees understand their part in fighting infection. Personal hygiene and hand washing must be taught and enforced.

Employee personal hygiene needs to be monitored on a daily basis by the supervisory staff. This will not necessarily be in writing, although disease monitoring of employees must be reported to the infection control nurse within the facility. Annual physicals are required by many state laws; these laws should be checked for the particular state to determine exactly what must be included.

Employees need to report any open wounds or sores and any contagious diseases they have. It is best to schedule these employees off duty until such time as they are noncontagious. For cuts or burns on fingers, gloves need to be worn to protect both the food and the worker. Gloves should also be worn for handling food, particularly food that is not going to be cooked after it is handled. Gloves on the serving line need to be on the hand that actually touches the food; the hand that touches the utensil does not need to be covered.

Infection control monitoring is another type of monitoring that is very helpful in ensuring that the food service department is maintaining the sanitary standards necessary. Periodic laboratory culturing of various surfaces and utensils is a safety check and an excellent demonstration for employee education concerning infection control.

Food needs to be heated to a temperature that will destroy bacteria and also any potential toxins that have been produced in the food by the bacteria.

Food Purchasing and Storage

Food purchasing involves buying, storing, inventorying, issuing, and managing food products and supplies. Storage areas need to be clean and dry as well as located outside high-traffic areas. To help eliminate theft, food and supplies should be issued and their use monitored.

When storing food, the department must follow the guidelines established by the state health department. These standards usually require that supplies be kept between 6 and 12 inches off the floor. The Joint Commission and the state health department both specify that chemical products must be stored separately from food products and clearly labeled. Dented cans must be removed from service in the event that they might be infected. In addition, dented cans should be returned to the vendor for a refund.

Freezer storage must be at −10° F to hold food at the zero-degree mark. Temperature gauges in refrigerators and freezers are required. Storerooms should be kept at normal room temperature. Store paper products separately from food products and unbox foods as quickly as possible in order to minimize pests, especially in southern climates.

☐ Program Evaluation

In order for any food service department to be a success, its staff must be in touch with the people it serves. This means patrons must be pleased with the food and service they receive. In the cafeteria, the cafeteria manager should talk with customers as they come through the line, food service workers should be pleasant and trained in guest relations techniques, and cashiers need to be aware of people's reactions and impressions as they pay for their food.

In the patient areas, the dietitians, the diet clerks, and the food service director are responsible for learning patients' reactions to their meals. Frequently, food service departments use surveys to obtain patient feedback. It is important that staff circulate during mealtimes and be in touch with patient suggestions (for improvement). Frequently, the difference between acceptance and rejection of hospital food can depend on the extent to which the food service department pays attention to the patients during their stay. This role cannot be overemphasized.

Monitoring of Food Preparation

In the food preparation area, temperature monitoring is critical. If the patient receives food at the wrong temperature, it is not only unappetizing but also a safety hazard.

Food not maintained in the proper range, 140° F or higher for hot food and 40° F or lower for cold food, is susceptible to bacterial growth. When held for even a short period of time, bacteria can grow very rapidly in infected food. Therefore, it is important that temperatures be monitored regularly throughout the day by meal and by serving. Sample patient trays need to be tested for temperature acceptability, and food on the service line needs to be evaluated by temperature checks at the start and end of the serving period. Delivery times must be monitored, as must the temperature of the food when it is delivered to patients. Corrective action must be immediate.

Hazardous food sampling is another way to ensure that food is available for testing if the need arises. Generally, bite-sized portions of foods that are considered potentially hazardous are set aside for 24 hours to see whether they are hazardous. Suspect foods are protein sources such as milk, puddings, meats, fish, poultry, eggs, as well as products that contain them, such as mayonnaise and chicken salad.

Another item to be monitored is the time of service. It is important to ensure that service times are within those prescribed by the health care facility. For example, if the tray line is to begin lunch service at 11:30 a.m. and finish at 12:30 p.m., but runs until 1:30 p.m., it significantly affects nursing services and other treatment areas within the hospital, as well as the timeliness of dish washing and food preparation in the kitchen.

Clinical Nutrition Monitoring

The Joint Commission requires health care facilities to have an ongoing QA program. The program's design should include ways to objectively and systematically monitor and evaluate the quality and appropriateness of patient care, as well as ways to improve patient care and resolve any identified problems.

To comply with this regulation, a food service department must have a clinical monitoring program in operation. This program is generally organized by the director or chief clinical dietitian or both, and it details standards of service, thresholds, and criteria for evaluation. The program also provides a plan for monitoring, evaluation, corrective action, and any follow-up measures that need to be done. Monitors should be established on the basis of high volume, high risk, or both, and for problem-prone aspects of clinical nutrition care.

Examples of clinical monitors are:

- Timeliness of nutrition intervention
- Appropriateness of nutrition intervention, such as diet order appropriate for diagnosis, long-term stay patient evaluations for diet tolerance/nutriture, identification of patients at nutritional risk, and incidence of premature readmittance of malnourished patients
- Appropriateness of internal nutrition therapy that includes products appropriate for diagnosis and patient tolerance to products
- Appropriateness of patient/family nutrition education, which can include drug or food interactions and appropriate instruction for patient condition and home environment

It is critical to have a mechanism in place for effectively analyzing and resolving day-to-day problems within food service operations. Problems need to be accurately documented and analyzed, and corrective action needs to be taken. Follow-up is also an important step in any plan of action to ensure that the problem has been corrected.

Effective management is high-quality management. Quality assurance is an integral aspect of that management, not a separate program.

☐ Summary

Ensuring high-quality food and service is the role the food service department plays in the overall function of the health care facility. Preparing timely meals that are nutritionally sound is just one way the department meets this goal. The department is also responsible for maintaining a budget, observing safety and sanitation rules, complying with federal and state laws and regulations, making nutritional assessments, and seeing that its employees follow good personal hygiene and health practices.

Leadership within the department is also an important element. Decisions must reflect the facility's desire to provide the best, most cost-effective care available and, at the same time, retain the morale of staff members.

☐ Bibliography

Joint Commission on Accreditation of Healthcare Organizations. *Accreditation Manual for Hospitals.* Oakbrook Terrace, IL: JCAHO, 1990.

Dietary Management Advisory, Inc. *Clinical Staffing Module-Food Service Management Evaluation and Analysis.* Wayne, PA: Dietary Management Advisory, 1990.

Appendix A

The Health Facility Development Process

Joseph G. Sprague

☐ Introduction

To be successful and competitive in today's rapidly changing marketplace, health facility planners need to address the enormous changes and trends confronting hospitals. The rising cost of health care, the changing nature of diseases, and the privatization of health care practice are major forces shaping today's planning efforts. With hospitalization costs averaging twice the consumer price index in the past several years, Americans are demanding more for their health care dollar.

These forces, as well as advancements in technology, have created rapidly changing environments within health care facilities. In addition to providing traditional care, hospitals must now be equipped to address other issues as well. Caring for AIDS patients, providing long-term services for trauma patients, and meeting the ever-growing needs of our aging population are just a few of these issues. And changes such as the growth of outpatient ambulatory care have significantly increased the need for nonhospital square footage compared with inpatient square footage.

The health facility development process should respond to these trends and offer alternative opportunities for appropriate solutions. When a facility decides to expand, by either building a new complex or remodeling existing areas within the facility, a well-organized plan should be developed that will not only meet the facility's current needs, but will also address future trends and demands.

☐ The Facility Development Team

A well-structured facility development team involves a multidisciplined approach. The team should include representatives from various departments within the hospital, such as administration, the board, medical staff, nursing services, and engineering, and planning and design specialists. In the early stages of development, either a hospital consultant or an architect specializing in health facility planning is key in structuring the team. Depending on the capabilities of the hospital, additional consulting members may be needed.

□ Preliminary Planning

One aspect of preliminary planning is developing a long-range plan of service for the entire health care facility. Services to be provided should be described in the facility's strategic plan, with specific goals and objectives outlined. The long-range plan should consider inpatient care, ancillary support, and outpatient services. Moreover, it should establish a framework for existing building and site use that will respond to future facility and program needs.

After the long-range plan and a facility development plan (described in the next section) have been developed, plans for specific project development should be established at various points in time. An immediate plan may be needed to address an upcoming licensing survey or a new physicians service, or to correct existing building deficiencies. An intermediate plan may be developed for a two- to five-year period in which the hospital implements specific objectives of the strategic plan. Examples of specific objectives could include the development of a medical office building, a new ambulatory surgery facility, or a cancer center.

□ Facility Development Plan

The facility development plan must be based on the long-range plan of service. A facility development plan involves three steps: investigation, evaluation, and planning. These steps work together to produce a development plan that can be effectively implemented.

Depending on the size of the facility, the three steps can be completed in 4 to 12 months. A 100- to 200-bed hospital may require four months (as shown in figure A-1). Moreover, a large teaching hospital with 1,000,000 or more square feet may require up to 12 months. However, for any size facility the steps are as follows:

1. *Investigation:* The purpose of this step is to review specific goals with all parties involved. During this organization and orientation process, communication is established and expectations should be documented. This phase identifies specific task analyses and each individual's area of responsibility throughout the development process. At the conclusion of this step, an agreement of project goals should be clearly understood.

   An integral part of the investigative process is site analysis. Current documentation should be reviewed to determine utility availability and capacity, site characteristics, and the proposed site's ability to accommodate growth and change. A site should be evaluated for its major visual access, as well as vehicular and pedestrian access. Perhaps the creation of a loop drive around the site should be considered to provide access from any direction. Land-use factors such as residential, agricultural, light industrial, or other zoning should be analyzed.

   Topography features, such as slope and drainage, create strong criteria for the location of building footprints. Making maximum use of topography for the separation of public and service access is important. Creating public access at the first level with service access at the garden level is an example. Equalizing access to both garden and first level eliminates undesirable basement spaces.

   Wind direction and sun angle are important considerations for orientation and building configuration. Other environmental factors, such as average temperature or rainfall, are also important.

2. *Evaluation:* This step should make maximum use of existing information by reviewing current documents such as statements of construction, record drawings, and facility management reports. In addition to the architectural, mechanical/electrical, and structural analysis for physical condition and code compliance, a functional performance evaluation should be done. Functional performance looks at

Figure A-1. Facility Development Plan for a 100- to 200-Bed Hospital

Activities	Project Months	1				2				3				4			
	Project Weeks	1	2	3	4	5	6	7	8	9	10	11	12	13	14	15	16
Investigation																	
Preview Planning Goals/Role/Trends		XXX															
Gather Statistical Data		XXXXXXXXXXXXX															
Area Survey			XXXXXXXXX														
Community Characteristics				XXX													
Health Characteristics				XXXXXXXXX													
Department Interviews				XXX													
Prepare Base Comprehensive Drawings			XXX			XXXXXXXXXXXXX											
Physical & Functional Facility Analysis		XXXXXXXXXXXXXXXXXXXX															
Site Analysis/Utilities Survey				XXX													
Evaluation																	
Work-Load Projections						XXX											
Space-Need Determination						XXXXXXXXXXXXX											
Future Site and Building Demands								XXX									
Manpower Needs						XXX											
Identify Options/Assess Priorities									XXX								
Planning																	
Master Site Plan										XXXXXXXXX							
Zoning Diagrams												XXXXXXXXX					
Schematic Plans														XXXXXXXXX			
Cost Estimates									XXX						XXX		
Final Report Publication/Rendering																XXXXXXXXXXXXX	
Review/Conference Sessions		*		*		*			*			*			*		*

both interdepartmental and intradepartmental relationships throughout the facility and optimizes those relationships.

Determining departmental locations and circulation flow through departments will enable the planner to increase the efficiency potential of the operation. For example, as supplies move throughout the facility, evaluation of the complete logistical support system is vital. An analysis of a supply item as it arrives at the loading dock should explain how it flows throughout the hospital to the patient bedside.

Site zoning is also important. Locating ambulatory care and inpatient zones within easy access of diagnostic and treatment departments optimizes patient care.

An in-depth departmental analysis is important to the facility development plan. Existing departmental operations, equipment, and personnel should be documented as they relate to the proposed future project. This process establishes specific growth objectives. This could be accomplished through the use of departmental questionnaires that outline individual departments' current and proposed requirements.

Reviewing the strategic plan and establishing specific identified goals will enable the team to prepare *concepts*, which are essentially ideas for implementation. For example, by looking at the site and locating the physician's office building, the emergency room entrance and the visitor/inpatient access can then be determined conceptually.

Determining departmental space requirements for both net and gross square foot projections can provide the approximate size for the proposed development. Alternative strategies of expanding and meeting both present and proposed needs of each departmental area, or contracting where appropriate, can be identified. Additionally, review of the site development studies can show the proposed department or building growth and changes in relationship to development concepts for future proposed projects.

3. *Planning:* The final step in developing a facility plan is to identify facility strategies, functional grouping (such as use of spaces that have specific relationships), and total circulation systems flow. A master zoning plan is typically developed to show a site plan including existing and projected proposed growth. The zoning plan must include specific parking requirements, in addition to roadway and vehicular traffic.

Prior to completion of the facility development plan, agreement must be reached by all parties involved in the process. Once everyone agrees with the development concept, a final presentation should be made to the board, the medical staff, and others who may not have been involved extensively to date.

☐ Steps in Health Facility Project Development

The traditional project development schedule, as shown in figure A-2, consists of a series of tandem steps that begin with programming and continue through design and also include construction documentation, bidding, and actual construction. Depending on the desired project schedule, various steps in the process can be overlapped to accelerate the completion date. These variations could include an accelerated design/construction phase, as well as accelerated and overlapped construction phases.

During the first step, the importance of a functional program cannot be understated. Most state licensure agencies require a functional program as a prerequisite to specific licensure requirements. The *functional program* describes the way in which the building works, including both intradepartmental and interdepartmental relationships. It describes general circulation and cooperation among various departments in the project.

Key to the functional program is a square-footage space program, which describes both net and gross square footages by room and department, as well as building net and gross square footages. The space program can be developed with the assistance of either a consultant or a hospital architect with programming expertise. The program effort involves extensive conferencing and data collection from every department within the hospital, and it is based on operational concepts, equipment requirements, and staffing. The space program is the first sizing of the project and is usually accompanied by a preliminary budget.

The next step, *schematic design,* typically starts with a departmental analysis involving alternative layouts, their relationship to each other, and how that relationship responds to the space program. This process is often referred to as a gaming activity (for example, charrette, esquisse-esquisse). Developing alternative departmental concepts will enable the team to do a series of optimizations, creating alternative concepts of arrangement. The overall departmental planning is then broken down into room-by-room plans. These room-by-room plans show the overall concept of each space within the facility and how each relates to adjacent spaces within the department.

At the same time the schematic design process proceeds, codes and standards research should be undertaken. The architect should search all pertinent local, state, and national codes and standards having an impact on the project. A clear understanding of various jurisdictional authority interpretations regarding code requirements is essential to avoid redesign and future problems. The American Hospital Association (AHA) publishes the *Health Facility Design Information Checklist* (ASHE Technical Document Series,

Figure A-2. Traditional Project Development Schedule

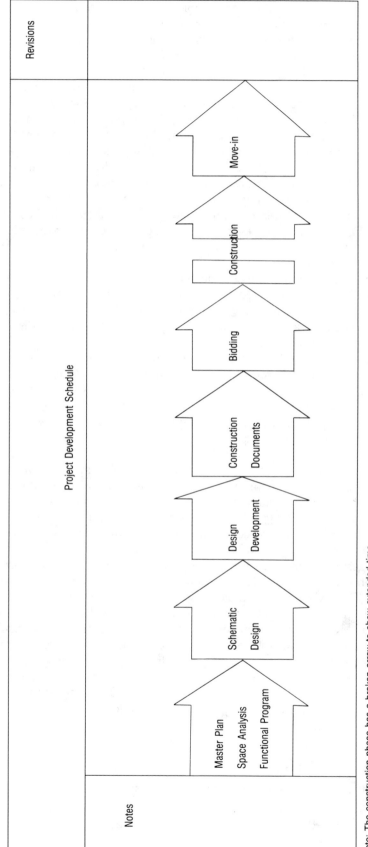

Note: The construction phase has a broken arrow to show extended time.

April 1988), which is a useful tool to complete code research in all areas—architectural, mechanical, electrical, plumbing, and fire protection.

Initial selection of all engineering systems is also developed during this process, including overall structural grids. Study models are good tools to communicate three-dimensionally to all members of the facility development team. As the project moves through schematic design, adding color and texture to the models further illustrates first impressions of the overall character and appearance of the facility.

Once a schematic concept is agreed upon, the team then moves into design development. Room data sheets are an important tool in design development that enable the designer to determine in detail all the elements that go into each room of the building. *Room data sheets* detail each room's architectural, acoustical, electrical, and mechanical elements as well as piping, equipment, and communications. Functional diagrams show appropriate furnishings and equipment placed in each room plan. Floor plans also show equipment and furnishings and are identified by key numbers, whereas reflected ceiling plans show lighting diffusers, returns, a ceiling grid, and ceiling-mounted equipment. Finally, a composite plan should be developed to evaluate and coordinate all the elements and reduce any conflicts.

As room data sheets are finished, detailed elevations of each exterior are completed. These elevations include detailed sections throughout the building.

Finally, the exterior image and appearance of the building are determined. An example of the exterior design can also be shown in model form to describe the overall appearance of the proposed project.

The longest phase in the design of the building is producing working drawings and specifications, commonly referred to as *construction documentation*. Every development of detail—architectural, mechanical, electrical, civil, and structural—is delineated in the construction documentation phase. Final fixed-equipment drawings, medical equipment drawings, and detailed cost estimates are prepared during this process. All decisions about medical technology and materials-handling systems are finalized and placed on the construction documents. Written specifications describing performance detail are then finalized and prepared for submission to qualified bidders, along with the working drawings.

Advertising for construction bids varies substantially from one project to the next. Contractors should be prequalified prior to receiving any bid proposal. Contractors base their bids on the plans and specifications, as well as any addenda included in the original construction document package. The selected contractor is then typically contracted directly by the owner to provide the construction.

The longest phase in the facility development process is the *actual construction* phase. Construction can last from several months to several years, depending on the size of the project. The architect has a major responsibility in construction administration. In fact, the American Institute of Architects (AIA) Standard Form of Agreement Between Owner and Architect provides approximately 20 percent of the architect's fee for administering the construction contract. Approximately half the architect's time during the construction phase is spent making periodic site visits. The other half is spent back in the office reviewing shop drawings and providing other administrative functions to support the construction progress. Owner-selected material substitutes and approvals are an integral part of the final decisions that complete the construction process.

☐ Design Philosophy

There are three key elements in design philosophy:

1. Form/function
2. Cost
3. Schedule

It is paramount that equal importance be placed on all these elements. If a beautiful, functional building is delivered within budget but six months late, the project is not likely to have been considered successful. Similarly, if the same building is delivered on time but 25 percent over budget, it is also likely to be considered unsuccessful. To ensure a successful outcome, both the architect and the owner must agree that these three elements are equally important.

The design process should consider operational and maintenance costs. The cost of designing and constructing a health care facility today equals the operational cost in 24 to 30 months. Expressed another way, capital cost equals operating cost in less than 2½ years. Therefore, it is paramount that any design compromise that contributes to increased operational costs must be avoided wherever possible.

Performing a staffing analysis is one way to design a facility with operational costs in mind. By modeling a nursing unit operation, for example, the required number of nursing personnel can be quantified. A nurse pushing a litter/gurney can go to an elevator lobby, push a call button, enter the car and go vertically one level, exit the car, and start down the hallway in approximately 60 seconds. That same nurse pushing the same litter/gurney can travel approximately 260 feet horizontally in that same 60 seconds (figure A-3). Although this exercise would indicate that horizontal design concepts can be much more efficient staffwise, other elements such as nursing unit size, distance from the nursing station, and building site limitations must be considered.

For this example, a nursing unit configuration evaluation must be done for each project under design. Numerous geometries and nursing unit layouts are possible. A decision to select one nursing unit design over another must take into account the nursing staff required to operate the unit. Time/distance measurements must be made that look at distances between the nursing station and patient rooms, the utility work core and the nursing station, and the utility work core and patient rooms.

Additional factors such as lineal feet of exterior wall, square feet of support area, square feet of unit area, area per bed, and overall circulation must be carefully analyzed. The design chosen must make maximum use of cost-effective technology and optimal staff utilization, and at the same time conserve energy and resources. (Figure A-4 on p. 145 shows a chart that ranks these concepts in order.)

Design decisions related to locating areas that have hard costs versus those that have soft costs are also important considerations. For example, hard-cost areas would be the high-labor, high-intensive, high-utility support departments (such as surgery, labor/delivery, radiology, and intensive care). Soft costs (such as the administrative area and support areas) are less expensive and could be relocated more easily, if necessary. This evaluation is very important when considering the need for adaptability and flexibility for future facility use. In fact, the evaluation is usually a requirement every hospital project confronts today.

For example, imaging services technically change more rapidly than probably any other service within the hospital. In just a few short years, imaging technology has gone from myelograms to CT scanning to magnetic resonance imaging. Imaging departments should always be placed near an outside wall so that as technology, growth, and expansion occur, space can be created to accommodate the imaging changes.

☐ Working with Restrictions on Capital

Before looking at specific tools and methods of controlling costs, it is important to review the project budget and how various costs are categorized. There are three distinct project budget costs that are quite often interchanged, but can be misleading: building cost, construction cost, and project cost.

Building cost is the building itself—the actual footprint of the construction, including all the architectural and engineering elements that go into the construction. To get to

Figure A-3. Time/Distance Diagram

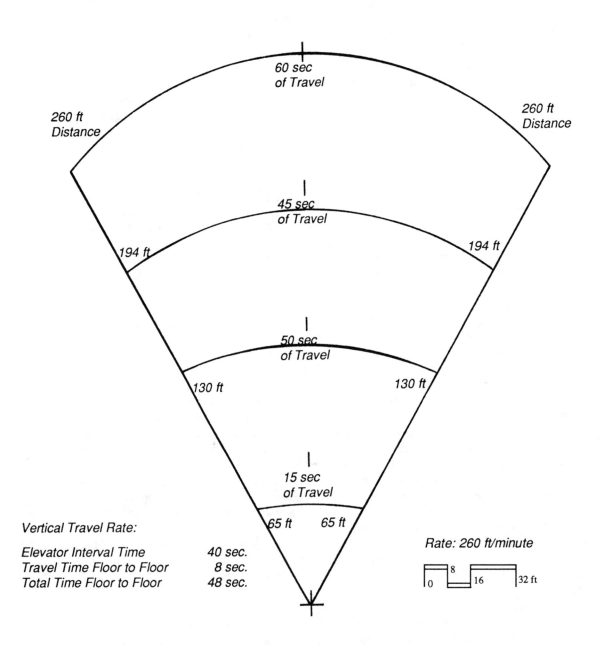

construction cost, fixed equipment and site development must be added to building cost. Fixed equipment can range from 15 percent to 35 percent of building cost depending on the amount of imaging and other high-cost technology items.

Site development typically ranges between 6 percent and 12 percent of building cost. Often a construction contingency of 5 percent to 10 percent is included in the construction cost.

Added to construction cost to arrive at total *project cost* are furniture and movable equipment, which can range from 15 percent to 35 percent of construction cost. Professional fees, including design, legal, permit, and filing fees approximate 10 percent, owner contingencies 5 percent, and administrative costs between 1 percent and 2 percent, to

Figure A-4. Nursing Unit Configuration Evaluation

Ranking by Category

Nursing Unit Floor Plan Configurations	Concept	Exterior Wall, Linear Foot	Support Area, Sq. Ft.	Unit Area Sq. Ft.	Area Per Bed, Sq. Ft.	Nurse Station to Patient Room Door (Average Distance)	Utility to Patient Room Door (Average Distance)	Nurse Station to Patient Room Door (Farthest Distance)
1	G	2	1	1	1	3	5	1
2	H	4	2	3	3	2	6	2
3	J	3	3	2	2	6	4	3
4	E	7	7	5	5	4	3	3
5	B	8	6	4	4	5	2	5
6	D	6	5	10	10	1	1	7
7	K	9	8	6	6	8	9	4
8	C	10	9	7	7	7	8	9
9	A	5	10	8	8	9	7	10
10	I	11	4	9	9	10	10	8
11	F	1	11	11	11	11	11	6

Note: This chart ranks each concept in order from best rating (1) to worst rating (11).

bring the project budget to project cost. Other elements of cost would include any land cost, off-site development costs, finance costs, and inflation. Typically, it is advisable to project the cost for inflation to the midpoint of construction. If the project construction schedule is 24 months, midpoint of construction would occur in 12 months.

An important tool in cost control during design is departmental cost factoring. Because health care facilities have a combination of uses such as restaurant, business, mercantile, hotel, and institutional, the cost per square foot can vary widely within the building. Departmental cost factors enable the designer to control the overall costs by understanding the cost of a square foot in each department. The cost for nursing service, for example, is typically 90 percent to 95 percent of the average square foot cost in the project. Diagnostic and treatment, on the other hand, is 120 percent to 130 percent. Other examples are public administration, 80 percent to 85 percent, and building services, 85 percent to 90 percent. Departmental cost factors can be generated for each department within the facility and should be used widely, particularly during the early stages of design.

Other cost control tools include life cycle cost analysis, where initial capital costs are balanced with maintenance and operational costs over the estimated life of the building. The AHA publication *Estimated Useful Lives of Depreciable Hospital Assets* (1988) can be helpful to the designer in making design decisions about buildings, building services equipment, fixed medical equipment, and major movable equipment. Another cost control tool, *cost balance,* looks at cost–benefit analysis through items such as energy conservation and value engineering. *Value engineering* is a process by which construction details can be suggested to reduce construction cost while maintaining design intent. Value engineering is an important tool, particularly where a construction manager is available during the design stages to provide recommendations for more cost-effective construction details and materials.

Besides these cost control tools, several other considerations affect the determination of costs. Designing for flexibility provides adaptive structures that can be modified through time. Adaptive flexibility requires weighing the cost today against future cost savings when changes will actually occur. Designing for disposability involves planned obsolescence to determine at what point in time the structure will be replaced. Selection of utility systems, materials, and finishes is often dependent on these assumptions.

☐ Schedule Control

A detailed work plan should be outlined and followed throughout the project to maintain schedule. Specific review sessions and conferences with hospital administration throughout the process will keep all parties informed and aware of any decisions that affect schedule.

Drawing control sheets, which show specific amounts of work accomplished versus specific amounts of work left, are important tools in keeping to schedule. They can be used by each discipline in the architectural and engineering area. As previously mentioned, acceleration of various stages of the project can be undertaken. Overlapping elements of the design and the construction phase is one way to accelerate the project. Combining these elements is also possible and often referred to as fast-track (see figure A-5).

☐ Design and Production Approach

Today's health facility development process involves a team approach. In-depth, predesign activities, including programming and planning, have a great effect on the outcome of the project. The administrator, project designer, project manager, and support staff should be led by experienced management in the development team. To ensure the project's acceptability, involvement of physicians, nurses, and other departmental people throughout the process is important.

The use of gaming activities, such as three-dimensional stacking zoning models and three-dimensional take-apart models, often assists in the communication between team members. For spaces that will be duplicated multiple times throughout the facility (such as patient rooms, intensive care units, or examination rooms), full-scale mock-up rooms can be used. Having nursing staff evaluate the details of rooms (such as headwall location, gases, receptacles, and lights) enables the design to reflect specific user requirements.

The use of computer-aided design and drafting is a sophisticated tool available during the design phase. Changes in lighting from day to night, color, texture, style, and overall environmental effect can all be simulated to help illustrate the finished design.

☐ Summary

As we look at the trends shaping today's health care environment, it is essential to understand the various components of the health facility development and construction process. In a health care setting, many factors must be taken into consideration before a facility can undertake a building project of any size. Because health care facilities are truly interdisciplinary in nature, the design effort must represent those multifaceted considerations.

As a health care facility undertakes any building project, building a strong team that supports and implements the strategic plan is essential to its success. Because the health care facility of tomorrow will go beyond traditional concepts, the planning and design process must allow and reflect anticipated changes and future opportunities.

Figure A-5.   Design/Construction Scheduling

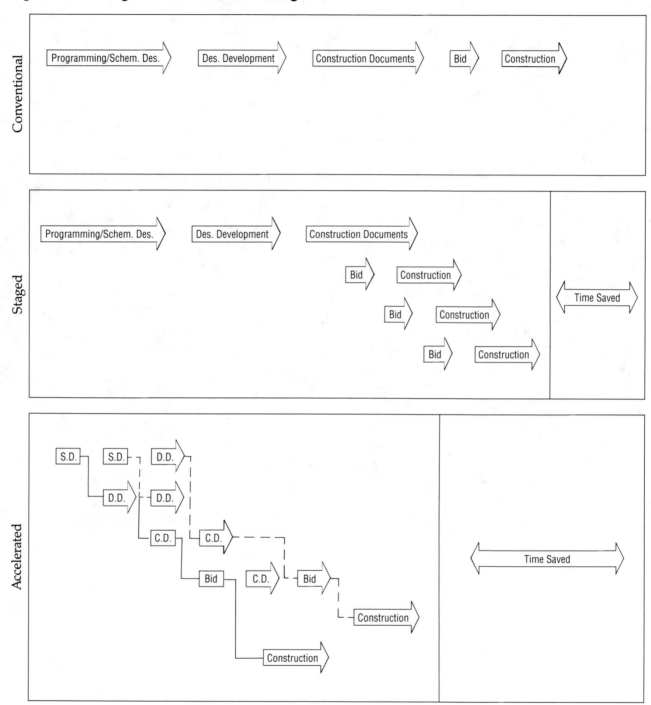

Appendix B

Architectural Influence on the History of Health Care Facilities

Leslie McCall Saunders

☐ The First Hospitals

The Greek and Roman civilizations were the first to have organized hospitals. The earliest Greek hospitals were built around 500 B.C. and were called *stoa*, the Greek word for "porch," or *asklepieia*, representing the god of dreams. These facilities were typically built adjacent to a temple or as a part of a temple complex. The temple and adjoining stoa were almost always located on a hill so that when the people worshiped and sought cures for their illnesses, they could be closer to the gods.

Obviously, treatment in the early Greek hospitals differed greatly from the treatment available in their modern-day counterparts. To receive a diagnosis, a "patient" would first go to the temple and sleep, and then report his or her dreams to the priests. In their turn, the priests interpreted the dreams and gave what was believed to be god-sent directions for treatment.

By the beginning of the Christian era, the Romans had established the *iatreion*, meaning "healthful place." Archeological evidence suggests that the iatreion was possibly an examination and treatment facility built adjacent to a private home, probably the physician's house.

Iatreia were generally quite small, usually no larger than two to three examination rooms, which suggests that their use was limited to the physician's private practice. Several ancient structures identified as iatreia seem to have adjacent guest rooms, although it is not clear whether these rooms were intended for patients or family friends and visitors.

The Romans also constructed *valetudinaria* (from the Roman word for "invalid"), military field hospitals that were modifications of the typical barracks-style housing used by the soldiers. These facilities were important to the military because most Roman soldiers were gladiators, slaves, or mercenaries who did not have homes to return to when they were sick or injured and who represented economic investments to be protected.

The medical staff at the valetudinarium cared for soldiers' combat wounds or locally contracted diseases. The facilities were constructed at the edge of the camp, adjacent to the crucifixion sites and graveyard.

☐ Hospitals in the Middle Ages

The Middle Ages (from A.D. 500 to 1500) witnessed the evolution of the hospital into a hospice (derived from the Latin word meaning "host"). Hospices were built adjacent to abbey churches and were operated by the parish brothers and sisters, who felt called by God to serve their fellowmen by providing them food, drink, housing, clothing, treatment, visitation, and even burial.

The typical hospice was more like an inn than a hospital. It contained two or more dining rooms, both private and public, and a mix of open wards and private rooms. Guests stayed until they died or were able to travel.

☐ Hospitals in the European Renaissance

It was during the European Renaissance (roughly the 14th through the 17th centuries) that the hospital evolved into a public service. Private medical care continued to be provided in the homes of wealthier patients, whereas poor or abandoned citizens were left to fend for themselves on the streets. As a public health measure, many communities created public houses, or *ospedali*. Again, these were generally run by the church.

These structures were often quite large and frequently housed up to 1,000 ill or dying residents. The architecture of these buildings was usually in the form of a cruciform, which was a symbolic reminder of the source of the funds, the care givers, and the mission of the facility (figure B-1). During this time, the chapel became part of the hospital because the hospital was no longer structurally attached to the church itself.

The cruciform hospitals contained many of the functional areas found in today's institutions: open wards, private rooms, staff quarters, kitchens, treatment areas, and storage and supply areas. Some of the facilities were single structures; others had several wings, or wards, joined together by courtyards.

The ospedali were generally built at the edge of town and, in many cases, housed both mentally and physically ill patients. Overcrowding was a problem; there were often scores of patients in one room and minimal sanitation.

☐ European Hospitals from the 1600s to the 1700s

Hospital patient care during the 1600s and the mid- to late 1700s changed little from the previous era. The changes that did occur during this period were architectural.

It was during this time that hospitals began to be designed along the *pavilion* concept, using independent structures (pavilions) connected by a common corridorlike link joining them to areas that provided support services (figure B-2). Each pavilion housed a different segment of the patient population, separating patients by age, sex, diagnosis, ethnic origin, and wealth.

The individual pavilions were smaller than the patient housing areas in the older, larger cruciform hospitals and had better cross-ventilation. Interestingly, the ventilation was intended to reduce odors more for the staff's well-being than the patients' health. Except for pavilions designated for wealthy patrons, where there might have been private rooms, the patient areas were open and housed as many as 60 individuals. In some cases, pavilions were up to three stories high.

☐ European Hospitals in the 1800s

The next significant change in hospital architecture came in the latter half of the 19th century, after the Crimean War. It was the conditions of patient care in this war that influenced these changes.

Figure B-1. Cruciform Hospital (Ground Floor Plan of Ospedale Maggiore, Milan, c. A.D. 1750)

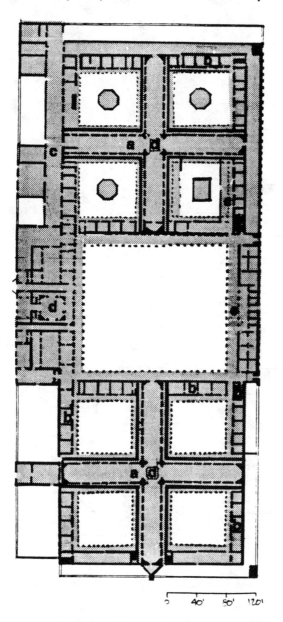

Note: a. Open ward areas.　b. Private room areas.　c. Support areas.　d. Chapel.　e. Public areas.

During England's war in the Crimea, a "nurse" named Florence Nightingale, against her family's wishes and contrary to society's acceptance, went to the battle areas and involved herself in the care of wounded and dying soldiers. It soon became obvious to her that climatic conditions made tent shelters inappropriate, so she appropriated farm and village houses to serve as makeshift hospitals. Because these buildings generally had several small rooms, the soldiers could be housed a few to a room, with each room having a medical attendant.

Nightingale observed that the health of these smaller groupings of patients did not deteriorate as rapidly and that the attendants were more easily able to monitor the patients than at the pavilion hospitals in Europe. Although Louis Pasteur had not yet published his findings on microbiology to explain the phenomena that Nightingale found, she

Figure B-2. Pavilion Plan Hospital (Site Plan, Johns Hopkins Hospital, 1885)

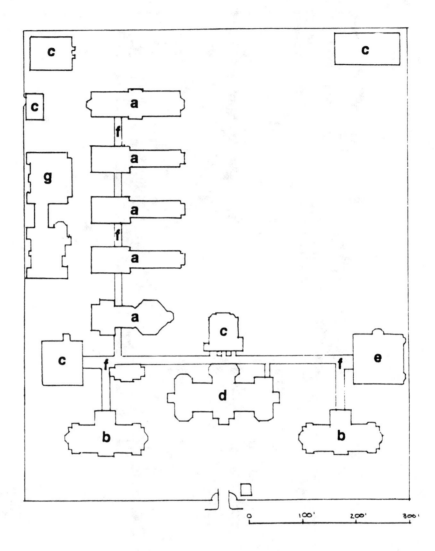

Note: a. Patient wards.   b. Paying-patient wards.   c. Support buildings.   d. Administration.   e. Nurses' home.   f. Connecting corridor.   g. Dispensary.

determined that ventilation, cleanliness, the placement of patients on beds instead of floors (to avoid contact with rats and insects), and a small patient population per room were instrumental in the recovery of patients who otherwise might have died.

Not only did Florence Nightingale's presence in this war give rise to the modern nursing profession, but her observations helped formulate a concept of hospital architecture that is still prevalent today: a small number of patients close to and easily monitored by a nurse (figure B-3). In many parts of the United States, the ward concept is still the only legally acceptable means of housing licensed critical care beds and is the design concept of preference for postanesthesia recovery rooms.

☐ Early American Hospitals

Although history of hospital architecture in the United States is of much shorter duration than in Europe, it is no less significant. The first structure in North America that

Figure B-3. Ward Plan Hospital (Second Floor Plan, Westminster Hospital, London, 1834)

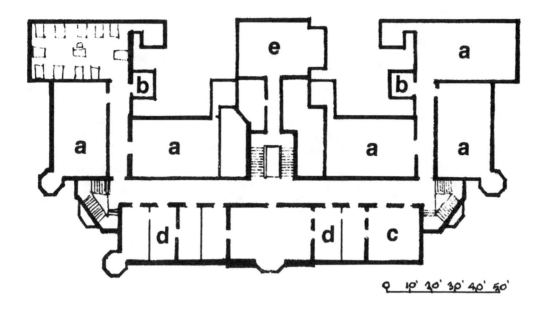

Note: a. 11-bed wards.   b. Washrooms.   c. Nurses' room.   d. Offices.   e. Chapel.

was specifically used for a hospital was built by the Spanish in Mexico City, in 1524. Large portions of the facility are still in use as the Jesus of Nazareth Hospital.

The earliest U.S. hospitals include the Quaker Alms House (1713) and Pennsylvania Hospital (1751), both in Philadelphia, and Massachusetts General Hospital (1782) in Boston. Although some treatment was provided at these institutions, their main purpose was to care for and house terminally or chronically ill citizens who were deemed "the worthy poor." Wealthy patients were treated and cared for at their homes or private sanitariums.

The first U.S. facility created specifically for patient care, teaching, and research was the New Haven Hospital. The research efforts of the hospital, namely the grave-robbing that was necessary to support anatomical research, drew a great deal of public criticism. However, the quality and success of patient care was widely lauded.

□ American Hospitals in the 1800s

By the mid-1830s, out of a total of between 100 and 120 American hospitals, 6 facilities were devoted to the care and treatment of patients. The majority were still places where patients went to die.

In 1880, there were 150 hospitals (facilities that primarily cared for the terminally ill), 20 nursing schools, and 4 medical schools. Hospital funding was almost always through philanthropic donations. Hospitals were managed by superintendents and governed by boards of directors who oversaw supply procurement, employee relations, patient admissions, and discharge. At this time there was no physician credentialing.

The transformation of the hospital from hospice to diagnostic and treatment center began in the late 1800s, coincidentally with and largely a result of the Industrial Revolution.

As medical education and knowledge advanced and long-distance communication improved, physicians were able to consult and exchange ideas with one another. During this time, the American Medical Association (AMA), founded in 1845, grew in numbers and stature as a self-policing, credentialing organization.

The Industrial Revolution not only brought about massive change in the workplace, but during this period there also was tremendous rise in industrial accidents and the need for surgical repair. To make surgery less traumatic for patients and at the same time permit longer surgical procedures, physicians had ether (1846) and nitrous oxide available to them.

In 1860, Louis Pasteur published his findings about microbiology, thus increasing the awareness of infections and their causes. In 1867, Joseph Lister published his theories on antiseptics, leading to the development of aseptic techniques. With the advent of these discoveries, the practice of surgery began to save more patients than it killed. Surgeons became respected practitioners, especially among fellow physicians, and were no longer thought of as butchers. During this time, it also became evident that well-equipped hospitals with trained surgical attendants and nurses could provide a better aseptic environment and a more efficient process for surgery than could surgeons/physicians working in patients' homes.

☐ American Hospitals in the Early 1900s

In the early 1900s, American physicians began admitting their private, wealthier patients to the wards and pavilion hospitals that had been created for that purpose. Generally, the hospital was perceived by society as an acceptable avenue for medical treatment and no longer as a "filthy, dirty hovel for the dying poor."

New anesthetics, procaine and novocaine (1905), came into use during this time. Hospital usage increased with the invention of radiology as a diagnostic tool (1915) and the formalization of microbiology, chemistry, and hematology as laboratory sciences. The membership of the AMA continued to grow, and by 1910, about half the physicians in the United States belonged to the AMA. By 1920, virtually all respected physicians belonged to this organization.

From the 1920s to the 1940s, medical specialties such as obstetrics and pediatrics evolved. The introduction of penicillin and sulfa drugs began the elimination of one of the leading killers of hospitalized patients—nosocomial (hospital-acquired) infections.

☐ American Hospitals in the Mid-1900s

The outbreak of World War II brought rapid advancements in medical technology. Not only were many new drugs and procedures introduced, but there was also a growth in radiology. Nuclear reaction and sonar led to nuclear medicine and ultrasound.

The successful use of antibiotics, field hospitals, and surgical repair increased the number of soldiers who lived through the war. As a result, American community hospitals and military hospitals were filled to capacity.

The Hill-Burton Act and Its Implications

To relieve overcrowding in hospitals, the Veterans Administration began its medical care services, and in 1946, Congress passed the Hill-Burton Act, which provided federal funds to communities for the construction of hospitals and medical care facilities.

The Hill-Burton Standards were created by the Health Care Financing Administration (HCFA) of the Public Health Service of the Department of Health, Education, and Welfare to assist planners and designers and ensure uniform quality and content in these facilities. These standards were regularly updated and eventually adopted by many states as the standards for construction of all hospitals (not just federally funded ones).

In 1965, the Hill-Burton Standards also became a requirement for licensing those hospitals qualified to receive Medicare and Medicaid reimbursement.

It is important to note that the Hill-Burton guidelines were established as minimum standards for construction. However, many states adopted portions of these standards as maximum standards. In an effort to reduce capital expenditures, many institutions constructed their facilities at the minimum standards. Consequently, many of today's hospital buildings are ill-suited for meeting today's complex, sophisticated, and space-intensive patient care needs.

The Hill-Burton program was responsible for the construction and expansion of the vast majority of the nation's community hospitals. Between 1950 and 1970, there was dramatic activity in hospital-related construction, ranging from additions to house new technologies to completely new facilities.

The hospitals during this period were almost totally inpatient-centered, making the patient *towers* the dominant features. These bed-towers were designed to accommodate as many beds per floor as practical. The *typical* hospital had beds on the upper floors and diagnostic and treatment facilities on the lower levels (figure B-4).

Prior to the 1950s, before air-conditioning was practical or affordable, hospitals were designed to maximize natural ventilation. As air-conditioning became more efficient, it was possible to create more interior rooms and maximize a building's site coverage.

Expansion in technology, services, and procedures increased the requirements for patient rooms, diagnostic and treatment spaces, and ancillary space. As hospitals became more sophisticated and larger, their management became more complex and, consequently, the space needed to house managers also increased.

☐ The Federal Government's Involvement in Health Care in the United States

From 1946 to 1965, the federal government's involvement in health care was limited primarily to financing hospital construction. The government had minor involvement in standards and accreditation and offered only limited health services through agencies such as the Veterans Administration, the Public Health Service, and the Indian Health Service.

In 1965, with the passage of legislation that created the Medicare and Medicaid programs, the federal government became directly involved with providing health services to virtually all segments of society. Although initially conceived as being small, contained programs, Medicare and Medicaid grew rapidly.

In the early 1970s, the government was faced with runaway hospital charges. It was determined that some of the cost increases might be contained if hospitals' capital expenditures were controlled. As a direct result of this belief, the Health Planning and Resource Development Act of 1974 (P.L. 93-641) was introduced and passed by Congress.

This new law created the system of certificates of need, which curtailed construction from 1974 through the mid-1980s. As a direct result of this law limiting construction expenses, many hospitals deferred modernization projects.

☐ The Impact of Modern Technology

As technology advanced, particularly in the 1960s and 1970s, the hospital became the "center of care, repair, and replace." Consequently, the architecture of the hospital changed to reflect (at least in space allocation) the growing importance of high-tech areas, such as diagnostics and treatment, over high-touch areas, such as inpatient care (figure B-5).

Figure B-4. Hospital Development during the 1950s and 1960s

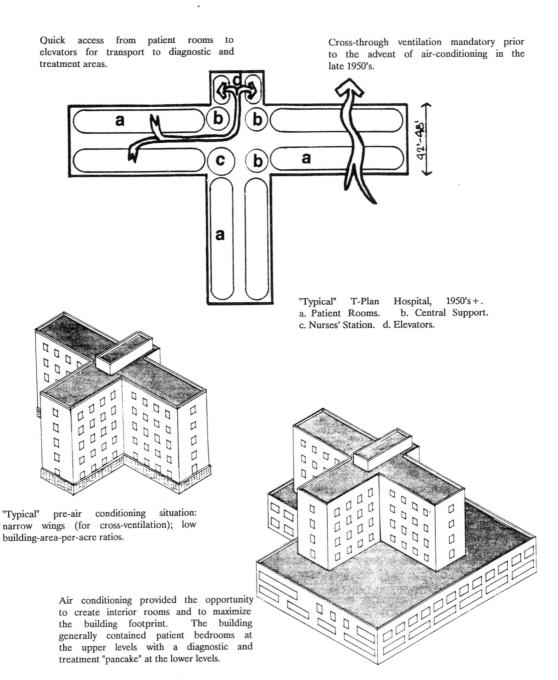

Quick access from patient rooms to elevators for transport to diagnostic and treatment areas.

Cross-through ventilation mandatory prior to the advent of air-conditioning in the late 1950's.

"Typical" T-Plan Hospital, 1950's +.
a. Patient Rooms. b. Central Support.
c. Nurses' Station. d. Elevators.

"Typical" pre-air conditioning situation: narrow wings (for cross-ventilation); low building-area-per-acre ratios.

Air conditioning provided the opportunity to create interior rooms and to maximize the building footprint. The building generally contained patient bedrooms at the upper levels with a diagnostic and treatment "pancake" at the lower levels.

The time line in figure B-6 on p. 158 provides an overview of the changes in hospitals and those in technology throughout history.

☐ American Hospitals in the 1980s

In the mid-1980s, the American hospital industry faced yet another challenge. The Tax Equity and Fiscal Responsibility Act (TEFRA) passed in 1983 mandated the reimbursement

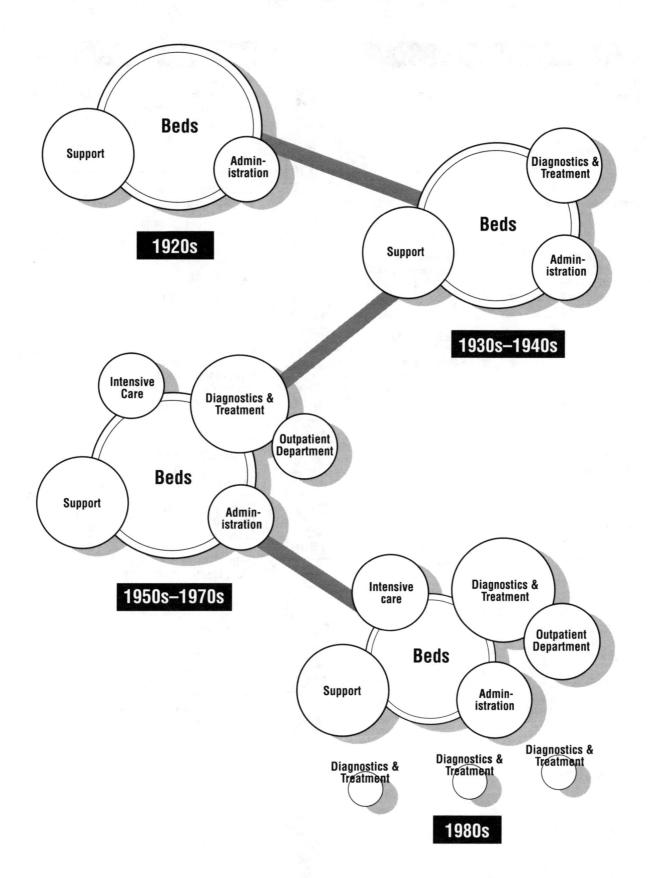

Figure B-6. Time Line Showing Relative Comparisons of Hospital Development to Technological Development

Hospitals		Technology
Roman iatreia		People die.
Greek stoa	c. 300 B.C.	Dying people make other people die.
		Some people can make
		other people well.
Abbey church	c. 900	
	1000	
		If it's green, cut it off.
Jesus of Nazareth Hospital	Mexico City, 1524	Surgery/"surgeons"
	1700	
Pavilion hospitals	England, 1700s	
Quaker Alms House	Philadelphia, 1713	
Pennsylvania Hospital	Philadelphia, 1751	
Massachusetts General Hospital	Boston, 1782	Ephraim McDowell
	1800	
Johns Hopkins	Baltimore, 1800	Ether, 1846
St. Louis De Paul	1828	Elizabeth Blackwell, 1849
Ward hospitals	Great Britain,	Crimean War, 1858
	U.S., 1860s	Louis Pasteur, 1860
		Flush toilet
American Medical Association	1845	Joseph Lister, 1867
First U.S. nursing school	1872	
	1900	
Private patients		Procaine/novocaine, 1905
Private insurance	Dallas, 1929	Marie Curie, 1915
		Surgery, radiology, microbiology
	1930	
Kaiser-Permanente system		Electron microscope
Blue Cross/Blue Shield		Obstetrics
		Penicillin
	1940	
Hill-Burton Act	1946	Sulfa
		World War II
		Nuclear reaction
		Human gestation period
	1950	
Joint Commission on		Korean War
Accreditation of Hospitals	1952	Nuclear medicine
MASH unit		Kidney transplant
		Radiation therapy
	1960	
Investor-owned hospitals	1960	Space program
First hospital computer	1960	Angiography/catheterization
Progressive patient care	1962	Heart transplant
Intensive care		
Medicare/Medicaid	1965	
	1970	
P.L.93.641 (HSAs, CONs)	1974	CAT
		Computer proliferation
		Monoclonal antibodies
	1980	
TEFRA/PPS/DRGs	1983	MRI
		Lithotripsy
		PET
"Recovery Hospital"		

of hospital inpatient services provided to Medicare and Medicaid recipients according to diagnosis-related groups (DRGs).

This DRG system, which was prospective pricing instead of cost-based reimbursement, encouraged or forced hospitals and physicians to minimize the length of stay for hospitalized patients and to treat more patients on an outpatient basis. Although outpatient usage had been increasing for some time, this new law and the private insurance industry's cost-containment efforts caused the percentage of outpatient treatments to rise rapidly.

Consumer Impact on Hospitals

After the passage of the TEFRA, hospitals were faced with a new architectural issue—how to accommodate the increase in mostly unaccompanied, ambulatory patients using hospital services. Adding to the dilemma was the increasing awareness among patients of their own health care needs. Patients not only began demanding second opinions but, as consumers, they expected the same convenience, options, and consideration they got when purchasing other goods and services. To meet these challenges, hospitals addressed these issues in several ways. Some located certain services off-site, others created ambulatory care centers (freestanding buildings or additions that housed many of the services most frequently used by outpatients), and still others reallocated space within their hospital to improve the outpatients' overall comfort.

Consumer pressure was also felt as hospitals began developing *health care malls,* the architectural answer to the consumer-oriented health care industry. In keeping with the mall philosophy, there were health care "boutiques" that offered women's centers, specialty clinics, imaging centers, outpatient surgery centers, and freestanding cancer treatment facilities.

Also during this time, American society experienced a wave of nostalgia. The architectural reflection of this nostalgia, called postmodernism, was characterized by the use of forms, colors, icons, and other elements of the classical eras. Consequently, hospital architecture in the 1980s began to show an awareness of image, which changed the stark simplicity that had traditionally characterized institutional facilities.

The End of Certificates-of-Need and Other Developments

During the mid-1980s, the federally mandated certificate-of-need (CON) system was discontinued. Many states did not reenact similar legislation, thus permitting hospitals to spend money on expansions they believed cost-effective or necessary. The states that chose to maintain a CON system generally loosened the restrictions on capital expenditures. As a result of this system no longer being in effect, there was a minor surge in construction activity across the country.

Many facilities wanted to upgrade their 20- to 30-year-old physical structures to keep pace with increased consumer awareness, advanced technology, continued popularity of outpatient-centered care, DRGs, and the need for increased productivity. Also, there was a rising awareness of the need for thoughtful master facility planning and of the interrelationships among facility planning, strategic planning, and marketing.

This set the stage for an interesting situation in the mid- to late 1980s. For numerous reasons, the nation's 6,000 hospitals found themselves operating with outdated physical plants and updated technology. In addition to the dramatic advances in health care technology, there were changes in the way care was delivered and in the patient base. The hospital care system had shifted from inpatient- to outpatient-centered care, and the typical inpatient was far more acutely ill than just 10 years ago.

Growing from these needs and trends has been the development of facility management, an area of concentration that has gained much attention and is now required study in many hospital administration academic curricula. By studying the history of the hospital, one can understand the forces that created the existing situations. Realizing that a hospital's facility is a reflection of the institution's culture and the community in which it is located helps one plan for the changes necessary to keep abreast of the rapidly advancing health care industry.

The hospital industry now sees itself as a business. It employs personnel, operates a physical structure, maintains equipment, and at the same time tries to make a profit. Institutional managers are increasingly aware of the need to improve their facility images to their patients and the community, and at the same time continue to promote productivity and efficiency within the facility.

☐ Bibliography

Allen, R. W., and Vonkardyi, I. *Hospital Planning Handbook.* New York City: John Wiley & Sons, 1976.

Califano, J. A., Jr. *America's Health Care Revolution: Who Lives? Who Dies? Who Pays?* New York City: Random House, 1986.

Coile, R. C., Jr. *The New Hospital: Future Strategies for a Changing Industry.* Rockville, MD: Aspen Publishers, 1986.

Lyons, A. S., and Pretrucelli, R. J. II. *Medicine: An Illustrated History.* New York City: Harry N. Abrams, 1978.

Porter, D. R. *Hospital Architecture: Guidelines for Design and Renovation.* Ann Arbor, MI: Health Administration Press, 1982.

Redstone, L. G. *Hospital and Health Care Facilities.* New York City: McGraw-Hill Book Co., 1978.

Rosenberg, C. E. *The Care of Strangers: The Rise of America's Hospital System.* New York City: Basic Books, 1987.

Snook, I. D., Jr. *Hospitals: What They Are and How They Work.* Rockville, MD: Aspen Publishers, 1981.

Thompson, J. D., and Goldin, G. *The Hospital: A Social and Architectural History.* New Haven, CT: Yale University Press, 1975.

Weeks, L. E., editor. *Health Care Systems in World Perspective.* Ann Arbor, MI: Health Administration Press, 1976.

Wheeler, E. T. *Hospital Modernization and Expansion.* New York City: McGraw-Hill Book Co., 1971.

Appendix C
List of Organizations

Agency for Toxic Substances and
  Disease Registry
1600 Clifton Road, N.E.
Atlanta, GA 30333
404/454-4630

American Hospital Association (AHA)
840 North Lake Shore Drive
Chicago, IL 60611
312/280-6000

American Industrial Hygiene
  Association (AIHA)
345 White Pond Drive
Akron, OH 44320
216/873-2442

American National Standards Institute
  (ANSI)
1430 Broadway
New York, NY 10018
212/354-3300

American Society for Healthcare
  Central Services Personnel
  (ASHCSP)
840 North Lake Shore Drive
Chicago, IL 60611
312/280-6160

American Society for Healthcare
  Environmental Services (ASHES)
840 North Lake Shore Drive
Chicago, IL 60611
312/280-6245

American Society for Hospital
  Engineering (ASHE)
840 North Lake Shore Drive
Chicago, IL 60611
312/280-6139

American Society for Hospital Food
  Service Administrators (ASHFSA)
840 North Lake Shore Drive
Chicago, IL 60611
312/280-6417

American Society for Hospital
  Materials Management (ASHMM)
840 North Lake Shore Drive
Chicago, IL 60611
312/280-6155

American Society for Industrial
  Security (ASIS)
1655 North Ft. Myer Drive, Suite 1200
Arlington, VA 22209
703/522-5800

American Society for Training and Development
600 Maryland Avenue, S.W., Suite 305
Washington, DC 20024
202/683-8100

American Society of Safety Engineers
850 Busse Highway
Park Ridge, IL 60068
708/692-4121

Association for the Advancement of Medical Instrumentation
3330 Washington Boulevard
Arlington, VA 22201
800/332-2264

Building Officials and Code Administrators International, Inc.
4051 West Flossmoor Road
Country Club Hills, IL 60477
708/799-2300

Centers for Disease Control (CDC)
1600 Clifton Road, N.E.
Atlanta, GA 30333
404/639-3311

Compressed Gas Association, Inc. (CGA)
1235 Jefferson Davis Highway
Arlington, VA 22202
703/979-0900

Emergency Care Research Institute (ECRI)
5200 Butler Pike
Plymouth Meeting, PA 19462
215/825-6000

Factory Mutual System
1151 Boston Providence Highway
Norwood, MA 02062
617/762-4300

Federal Communications Commission (FCC)
Washington, DC 20554
202/245-6000

Federal Emergency Management Agency
P.O. Box 70274
Washington, DC 20472
202/646-2500

Federal Register
Superintendent of Documents, U.S. Government Printing Office
Washington, DC 20402
202/783-3238

International Association for Healthcare Security and Safety
P.O. Box 637
Lombard, IL 60148-9942
708/953-0990

International Conference of Building Officials
5360 South Workman Mill Road
Whittier, CA 90601
213/699-0541

International Fabricare Institute (IFI)
12251 Tech Road
Silver Spring, MD 20904
301/622-1900

Joint Commission on Accreditation of Healthcare Organizations (JCAHO)
One Renaissance Boulevard
Oakbrook Terrace, IL 60181
708/916-5600

National Association of Institutional Laundry Managers (NAILM)
2130 Lexington Road, Suite H
Richmond, KY 40475
606/624-0177

National Fire Protection Association (NFPA)
Batterymarch Park
Quincy, MA 02269
800/344-3555

National Institute of Occupational Safety and Health (NIOSH)
4676 Columbia Parkway
Cincinnati, OH 45226
513/533-8236

National Restaurant Association
311 First Street, N.W.
Washington, DC 20001
202/331-5900

National Safety Council
444 North Michigan Avenue
Chicago, IL 60611
312/527-4800

National Sanitation Foundation
3475 Plymouth Road
Ann Arbor, MI 48106
313/769-8010

**Occupational Safety and Health
Administration (OSHA)**
U.S. Department of Labor
Washington, DC 20402
202/523-8063
(*Note:* OSHA regional offices are listed
in table 6-1 in chapter 6.)

Practicioner Reporting System
United States Pharmacopoeia
12601 Twinbrook Parkway
Rockville, MD 20852
800/638-6725

**Southern Building Code Congress
International, Inc.**
900 Montclair Road
Birmingham, AL 35213
205/591-1853

Underwriters Laboratories
333 Pfingsten Road
Northbrook, IL 60062
708/272-8800

U.S. Department of Transportation
400 7th Street, S.W.
Washington, DC 20590
202/366-4000

**U.S. Environmental Protection Agency
(EPA)**
Office of Solid Waste and Emergency
Response
Washington, DC 20460
202/382-4700
(*Note:* EPA regional offices are listed in
table 6-2 in chapter 6.)

**U.S. Food and Drug Administration
(FDA)**
5600 Fishers Lane
Rockville, MD 20857
301/443-1544

**U.S. Nuclear Regulatory Commission
(NRC)**
1717 H Street
Washington, DC 20555
202/492-7000

Index